Understanding Suicide

CW00848202

Understanding Suicide

A Sociological Autopsy

Ben Fincham
University of Sussex, UK

Susanne Langer
University of Liverpool, UK

Jonathan Scourfield
Cardiff University, UK

Michael Shiner
London School of Economics and Political Science, UK

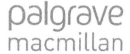

First published 2011 by
PALGRAVE MACMILLAN

Palgrave Macmillan in the UK is an imprint of Macmillan Publishers Limited,
registered in England, company number 785998, of Houndmills, Basingstoke,
Hampshire RG21 6XS.

Palgrave Macmillan in the US is a division of St Martin's Press LLC,
175 Fifth Avenue, New York, NY 10010.

Palgrave Macmillan is the global academic imprint of the above companies
and has companies and representatives throughout the world.

Palgrave® and Macmillan® are registered trademarks in the United States,
the United Kingdom, Europe and other countries

ISBN 978-1-349-36891-4   ISBN 978-0-230-31407-8 (eBook)
DOI 10.1057/9780230314078

This book is printed on paper suitable for recycling and made from fully
managed and sustained forest sources. Logging, pulping and manufacturing
processes are expected to conform to the environmental regulations of the
country of origin.

A catalogue record for this book is available from the British Library.

Library of Congress Cataloging-in-Publication Data

Understanding suicide : a sociological autopsy / Ben Fincham ... [et al.].
    p. cm.
    Includes bibliographical references and index.

    1. Suicide–Sociological aspects. I. Fincham, Benjamin.
    HV6545.U38 2011
    362.28–dc22   2011013744

10   9   8   7   6   5   4   3   2   1
20 19 18 17 16 15 14 13 12 11

Transferred to Digital Printing in 2012

Contents

List of Figures and Tables   vi

Acknowledgements   vii

Chapter 1   Introduction   1

Chapter 2   The Sociology of Suicide – A Critical Appreciation   7

Chapter 3   What is a Sociological Autopsy?   38

Chapter 4   Suicide Case Files as Sites of Identity Creation   65

Chapter 5   Suicide Notes as Social Documents   85

Chapter 6   Repertoires of Action   107

Chapter 7   When Things Fall Apart – Suicide and the   133
            Life-Course

Chapter 8   Lessons for Prevention   168

References   187

Index   200

List of Figures and Tables

Figures

7.1 Number of Suicides in England and Wales by   146
    Age and Sex (2008)
7.2 Rate of Suicide in England and Wales per 100,000   147
    by Age and Sex (2008)
7.3 Health Status by Age (percentage)   157

Tables

3.1 Para-phrased Summary of Evidence about   59
    Jane (Case 42)
7.1 Family and Interpersonal Relationships   150
7.2 How the Social Circumstances of Suicide Vary by Age 152
    and Sex (Cramer's V)
7.3 Relationship Breakdown and Problems Related to   155
    Children by Age (percentages)

Acknowledgements

Chapters 3, 4 and 7 draw on material which originally appeared in the journal articles listed below. We thank Blackwell and Elsevier publishers for permission to draw on this work:

Langer, S., Scourfield, J. and Fincham, B. (2008) 'Documenting the quick and the dead: A study of suicide case files in a coroner's office'. *Sociological Review* 56(2): 293–308.

Shiner, M., Scourfield, J., Fincham, B. and Langer, S. (2009) 'When things fall apart: Gender and suicide across the life course'. *Social Science and Medicine*, 69: 738–46.

Scourfield, J., Fincham, B., Langer, S. and Shiner, M. (2010) 'Sociological autopsy: An integrated approach to the study of suicide in men'. *Social Science and Medicine*, on-line publication ahead of print, doi:10.1016/j.socscimed.2010.01.054.

The research was funded by Economic and Social Research Council grant RES 576 25 5011. The authors would like to record their gratitude to the staff at the Coroner's office for their help with the study.

1
Introduction

Suicide is – arguably – a uniquely fascinating topic. In the aftermath of a suicide, those who knew the deceased always dwell on the question 'why?' This is in part because the reasons for a suicide are never really knowable, the most obvious witness being dead. It is also perhaps because the non-suicidal majority who put considerable effort into living find it very hard to understand the desire to end life. Perhaps news of a suicide also reminds us of our own frailty. Encountering death, according to Peter Berger ([1967] 1990), causes us to radically question 'the taken-for-granted "business-as-usual" attitude in which one exists in everyday life' (p. 43).

Suicide has a very important place in the history of sociology, because of Durkheim's (2002 [1897]) famous study of the social context of an ostensibly individual act, which was ground-breaking in terms of social scientific theory and method. Suicide is still a standard topic on introductory undergraduate sociology modules, as it remains a powerful illustration of competing paradigms, typically with reference to Durkheim, Douglas (1967) and Atkinson (1978). Our bold aim in this book is to make a new contribution to this classic sociological debate. We take a fresh look at sociological classics and also engage with new data. We assert the value of sociological research on *individual* suicides; we illustrate some ways in which qualitative and quantitative data can be integrated; and we navigate the dual paradigms of objectivism and constructionism. We aim for a methodological and empirical reinvigoration of the sociology of suicide.

We call our approach a 'sociological autopsy' in conscious mimicry of the psychological autopsy studies which are often carried out by medical and psychological suicide researchers. The empirical basis of the book is a study of 100 suicide case files from a coroner's office in the UK. The sample includes men and women of all ages and from diverse backgrounds. The research was funded by the UK Economic and Social Research Council (ESRC) and was based in the Cardiff 'node' of the National Centre for Research Methods – Qualitative Research Methods in the Social Sciences: Innovation, Integration and Impact (Qualiti).

In addition to methodological innovation, several important substantive themes are developed in the book. The gendered character of suicidal behaviour is one of these; especially important since around three times as many men kill themselves as women in the UK (and a similar trend is found across most of the world). Suicide across the life-course is another theme, theorised in relation to the social bond and the importance of attachment. The importance of intimate relationships is another thread which runs through the book. Some chapters take a more constructionist approach to the data, exploring the social processes involved in the construction of suicide files, while others lean towards an objectivist reading. And at the end of the book a chapter focuses on the potential implications of qualitatively-driven research for policy and practice in suicide prevention.

Hjelmeland and Knizek (2010) found that only 2.8 per cent of all articles published in the three international suicide research journals in 2005–7 were based on qualitative research. There are many reasons for the marginality of qualitative work on suicide to date. One is that the suicide research field is dominated by psychiatry and psychology. The prominent innovations in recent years have been in genetics research and neuroscience, so suicidology has arguably been becoming more rather than less medical in orientation. The 'psy' sciences are clearly dominated by quantitative approaches and many of the influential researchers in these fields would be positively hostile to qualitative approaches. (It should be noted that the opposite hostility tends to lurk in British schools of sociology.) Sociology is in fact only a bit-part player in terms of worldwide suicide research. Agerbo, Stack and Petersen (2009) found that out of over 30,000 academic papers on suicide published since 1980 (and in the Institute of Science Information database) there were only 400 which could be categorised as sociological. As Stack's (2000a and 2000b) review papers show, where there is sociological research on suicide it also tends to be quantitative. This is in part because most of it comes from the USA, which has a strong tradition of quantitative 'professional sociology' (Burawoy, 2005), that is, skilled analysis of large data sets to test hypotheses related to sociological theory. This is a very different tradition from the critical, and increasingly cultural, sociology which is dominant in the UK. Much recent and contemporary sociological research on suicide follows in the Durkheimian tradition of quantitative research on suicide rates so there is relatively little individual-level data (and where there are individual-level data they tend to be exclusively quantitative).

Despite the marginal position of sociology within the wider field of suicide research, the best-known sociological approach to the topic, that of Durkheim (2002 [1897]), has been very influential within suicidology and is still very frequently used in contemporary studies. Durkheim's idea was to study the social context of an ostensibly individual act by examining associations between suicide rates and various social factors (such as integration and regulation). This approach has generated considerable debate. Douglas (1967), in an important contribution, argued in opposition to the Durkheimian tradition for a Weberian emphasis on the subjective meanings of suicidal behaviour to social actors. Although his book is often cited now as an important contribution, Douglas's research agenda was not taken up to any noticeable extent. Atkinson (1978) made another important contribution to the sociology of suicide, in deconstructing through careful ethnomethodological research the reliance of published suicide rates on common sense reasoning by coroners in making their verdicts. Atkinson's conclusion was that we can only address suicide prevention through sociological research to a very limited extent, given the problems that there are with knowledge about suicide cases.

These classic contributions, along with Cavan's (1965 [1928]) are discussed in detail in Chapter 2. This chapter sets the context for the rest of the book by summarising some of the main debates about suicide within sociology. It focuses on Durkheim, Cavan, Douglas and Atkinson and concludes by considering the implications of Giddens's theory of structuration and Bourdieu's social praxeology. Chapter 3 justifies, in some detail, the research approach on which the book is based – the sociological autopsy of individual suicides. There is discussion of the qualitatively-driven mixed methods approach and also the use of dual paradigms. Some initial illustrations are offered of the kinds of insights a sociological autopsy can provide, with particular reference to the gendered dimension of suicide.

Chapters 4 and 5 take a broadly constructionist approach. In keeping with recent critiques of literature on the body and the life-course, the argument of Chapter 4 is that social identities can, to a certain extent, be constructed post-mortem and in the absence of a living body. This case is made with reference to the sociological autopsy study and it draws on ethnographic approaches to the study of documents. There is discussion of some of the diverse arte-facts in the coroners' files: medical reports, witness statements and suicide notes. The identity work revealed in these sources is as much about the living as the dead and is especially bound up with the process of avoiding blame. Chapter 5 turns to the suicide notes that were part of over 40 per cent of case files studied. Suicide notes are highly charged documents full of emotions and ambiguities. We pay attention to the notes' material aspects as well as their content and explore them with a focus on notions of agency, autonomy and the importance of relationships. Suicide notes tend to be the last artefacts created by the deceased and in the inquest files they were the only type of document written by the deceased, rather than about them. Suicide notes therefore constitute an immensely valu-able resource to study the explanations and motivations of those about to take their life. While Chapters 4 and 5 take a more con-structionist approach than Chapters 6 and 7, all these empirical chapters point to the importance of relationships to a sociological understanding of the context of suicide.

The search for causality has turned out to be challenging for suicido-logy. The isolation of variables associated with suicidal behaviour does not always sit comfortably with a consideration of the com-plexity of individual cases. Chapter 6 highlights the limitations of the stimulus-response model of causation and makes the case for a more nuanced psychosocial approach. Through the idea of 'repertoires of action' the argument is made that individual suicidal events can best be understood by the changing relationship people have to their perception of their situation, the perception they have of themselves and the perception they have of what people like them – in their situation – might reasonably do. In Chapter 6 we have focused on providing thick description within the framework of repertoires of action and a more fully theorised perspective on suicide is developed in Chapter 7.

Chapter 7 presents our quantitative analysis and provides a more objectivist reading of the data. This analysis compliments and extends the preceding qualitative work by showing how suicide and its associated meanings and motivations are structured by broader social relations, particularly those associated with the life-course. Drawing on official statistics and data from the sociological autopsy we argue that the relative vulnerability of 'young' men to suicide is often exaggerated and that insufficient attention is paid to the diverse social circumstances of suicidal men and women across the life-course. Bivariate analysis of the 100 cases reveals patterns of suicide that can be seen to map on to conventional features of a socially structured life-course, with young people in crisis, mid-life gendered patterns of work and family and older people in decline. Cases involving the breakdown of intimate relationships are subject to further qualitative analysis because they are central to gendered patterns of suicide and because they illustrate the key emerging themes of attachment and the workings of the social bond. Where relationship breakdown seems to have been the principal trigger, we highlight the role of punishment, over-dependence, sexual jealousy and separation from children.

Chapter 8 concludes the book, first by critically assessing its contribution to research and theory on suicide. There is then a discussion of some key documents which underpin suicide prevention strategy in the UK. Practice implications of the theoretical and pragmatic observations made throughout the work are discussed in relation to a range of relevant professions.

The book's authors have a range of different academic backgrounds within the social sciences and humanities. Coincidentally, all of us studied History as undergraduates. Ben Fincham is now primarily a sociologist, with a particular interest in work. Jonathan Scour-field is a social work academic with a particular interest in gender. Michael Shiner is a criminologist with a background in research methodology and a recent developing interest in psychoanalysis. Susanne Langer is an anthropologist, albeit one who has worked in research groups which are more focused on sociology and on medicine. We note this diversity to explain the use of concepts from outside of sociology or at least outside of the more predictable field of medical sociology. We hope our combination of interests leads to an exploration of the potential for creative new social science approaches to an old topic.

2
The Sociology of Suicide – A Critical Appreciation

There is currently little dialogue between sociology and suicide studies, which may seem surprising given the central role that Durkheim's (2002 [1897]) *Suicide* played in the construction of sociology as a distinct discipline. Although a series of influential studies followed in the wake of Durkheim's, emanating from various schools of thought, suicide has ceased to be of much interest to mainstream sociology. While contemporary sociologists have little to say on the subject, suicidology is dominated by various disciplines allied to medicine, including psychology, psychiatry and epidemiology. In this chapter, and in much of what follows, our aim is to re-engage with, and hopefully reinvigorate, the sociology of suicide. We begin here by reviewing four key studies that have been selected to illustrate the main sociological perspectives that have been applied to the subject. We start, inevitably, with Durkheim, before moving onto the work of Cavan (1965 [1928]), Douglas (1967) and Atkinson (1978). Coverage of these studies is followed by a brief review of more recent developments, which leads into a broader discussion of some key epistemological and ontological questions that we believe are fundamental to any sociology of suicide. Our answers to the questions we pose are rooted in a form of principled pragmatism: that is, we seek to transcend the unhelpful oppositions and dichotomies that have tended to dominate sociology, such as those that are often drawn between subjectivism and objectivism, social structure and human agency, the individual and the collective (Jenks, 1998). In so doing, we hope to move towards a more rounded analytical approach.

A retrospective

The study of suicide has a long history, stretching back several centuries. Early writers on the subject tended to focus on the moral implications of the act, but such considerations were displaced towards the end of the eighteenth century when apparently rapidly rising rates of suicide across much of Europe stimulated more objective concerns about the determinants of suicide. 'In terms of sheer bulk of material', suicide proved 'one of the most discussed social problems of the nineteenth century' (Giddens, 1965: 4). Considerable attention was given, at this time, to explaining differential suicide rates in terms of racial and climatic factors, while it was generally taken for granted that there was a close relationship between suicide and mental disorder. The publication of Durkheim's *Le Suicide* in 1897 represented a watershed. This work not only signalled the arrival of a distinctly sociological approach to the study of suicide, but was also a landmark in the development of sociology more generally. According to a volume honouring the centennial of its publication, *Le Suicide* is widely considered to be one of the three most important works ever written in the social sciences (Lester, 1994).

The studies featured below are all seminal works in the sociology of suicide and represent a range of distinct traditions or schools of thought. As well as providing historical 'depth' (Giddens, 1965), these studies are of considerable contemporary interest, not least because they identify a series of themes and controversies that remain central to our understanding of suicide. More than this, the works of Durkheim, Cavan, Douglas and Atkinson remind us that, for all that has changed, considerable continuities remain, both in relation to the nature of suicide and the way in which it is understood. By paying attention to such work we hope to see further than we might otherwise have done and to avoid the pit falls of chronocentrism, whereby disciplines lose sight of their past, only to get caught up in a recurring cycle of reinvention and new beginnings (Rock, 2005).

Emile Durkheim (2002 [1897]) *Suicide: A Study in Sociology*

Durkheim's study of suicide was formulated in the midst of a broader struggle to establish sociology as a recognised academic discipline and was explicitly geared towards vindicating the approach he advocated in *Rules of Sociological Method*. According to Durkheim the 'basic proposition that social facts are objective', which 'we consider the fundamental principle of the sociologic method' 'finds a new and especially conclusive proof in moral statistics and above all in the statistics of suicide' (2002: 274). Among the principle targets of Durkheim's polemic were those, such as Esquirol, who advocated the psychiatric thesis, arguing that mental disorder was the main cause of suicide, and those, such as Tarde, who offered a competing conception of sociology based on the study of micro-interactions among individuals (Giddens, 1965). Condemning such thinking as 'reductionist', Durkheim insisted that: 'Sociological method as we practice it rests wholly on the basic principle that social facts must be studied as things, that is, as realities external to the individual' (2002: xxxvi). Suicide was well suited to illustrating this point because it appears to be wholly 'an individual action affecting the individual only' (2002: xliv). If such an 'obviously' individual phenomenon can be shown to have an external reality then the general proposition has been proven beyond doubt. In developing his thesis, Durkheim did not limit himself to delineating a sociological analysis of suicide, moreover, but proceeded 'as if the role of psychology in the explanation of suicide would be a subordinate one' (Giddens, 1965: 5).

For Durkheim then, sociology should focus on suicide rates rather than individual cases, which should be left to psychology. The suicide rate of a society or community, he maintained, 'is not simply a sum of independent units, a collective total, but is itself a new social fact *sui generis*, with its own unity, individuality and consequently its own nature' (2002: xliv). Disregarding the individual, Durkheim sought 'directly the states of the various social environments...in terms of which the variations of suicide occur', only then returning to the individual to see 'how these general causes become individualized so as to produce the homicidal results involved' (2002: 104). Using official suicide records, covering France and other parts of Europe, Durkheim rejected inherited insanity, psychological imitation, race and various 'cosmic' factors as possible determinants of the distribution of suicide, whilst also noting that certain categories of people are more likely to commit suicide than others. Suicide rates, for example, were found to be higher among men than women, Protestants than Catholics or Jews, the wealthy than the poor and single people than married people. It was also noted that suicide rates tend to increase during times of economic change or instability, but decrease in times of war. Most, if not all, of these patterns had already been documented by other writers and Durkheim took much of his material from the likes of Legoyt, Morselli and Wagner. Consequently, the originality of *Suicide* lay not in its empirical analysis, but in the insistence on developing a coherent sociological theory to explain what had already been observed by others (Giddens, 1965).

Having rejected the main explanations of the time, Durkheim insists that the distribution of suicide is determined by aspects of social structure. Suicide rates, he notes, vary between societies, but show considerable consistency and regularity over time, prompting the conclusion that: 'At each moment of its history, therefore, each society has a definite aptitude for suicide' (2002: xlv). This aptitude, Durkheim argues, is a function of the 'collective conscience' or the shared beliefs and sentiments that bind people together and from which each individual conscience draws its moral sustenance. The workings of the collective conscience are, therefore, said to be tied up with the nature of social solidarity and the social bond: 'Man's characteristic privilege is that the bond he accepts is not physical but moral; that is, social. He is governed not by a material environment brutally imposed on him, but by a conscience superior to his own, the superiority of which he feels' (2002: 213). Based on his statistical analysis, Durkheim identifies three main types of suicide: egoistic, anomic and altruistic; which he attributes to different types of social structure. Additionally, the sharp increases in the suicide rate that were apparent during the nineteenth century are considered symptomatic of a deep crisis in modern society; one that was rooted in the weakening of the collective conscience and the growth of individualism. As the predominant forms of suicide in modern society, moreover, egoistic and anomic suicide are considered to be products of a low level of 'integration' and a dearth of regulative norms respectively.

Egoistic suicide, insists Durkheim (2002: 173), 'well deserved' its name:

> Egoism is not merely a contributing factor in it; it is its generating cause. In this case the bond attaching man to life relaxes because that attaching him to society is itself slack. The incidents of private life which seem the direct inspiration of suicide and are considered

its determining causes are in reality only incidental causes. The individual yields to the slightest shock of circumstances because the state of society has made him a ready prey to suicide.

Within this category of suicide, Durkheim discusses the role of religious affiliation, marriage and the family as well as political and national communities. Religion, he argues, reduces the suicide rate, not because of specific teachings or prohibitions, but because it constitutes a society built on common beliefs and practices. The more numerous and strong these 'collective states of mind', the stronger the integration of the community and the greater the protection offered to its members. Protestantism was judged to be less consistent than Catholicism or Judaism in this regard due to its emphasis on religious individualism and free inquiry, with the result that it created 'a less strongly integrated church' (2002: 114) and its moderating effect on suicide was reduced. The taste for free inquiry, Durkheim insists, can only be aroused if accompanied by a taste for learning, so that intellectual activity increases with the suicide rate due to the influence of religious disorganisation: 'Man seeks to learn and man kills himself because of the loss of cohesion in his religious society; he does not kill himself because of his learning' (2002: 123).

The protection offered by society is also said to be evident in relation to family and political life. Thus, Durkheim argues, egoistic suicide can be seen where there is slight integration of the individual into the family, so that the greater the density of the family the greater the immunity to suicide. The individual characteristics of the spouse are considered unimportant in explaining the suicide rate, which is said to depend upon the structure of the family and the roles played by its members. With the proviso that 'too early' marriages have an aggravating influence, Durkheim identified a general 'law' that married persons of both sexes benefit from a 'coefficient of preservation' in comparison with unmarried persons. This 'immunity of married persons', he goes on to show, has little to do with marriage – or 'conjugal society' – *per se* and is due largely to the influence of 'family society' (2002: 146):

...the fact remains that the family is the essential factor in the immunity of married persons, that is, the family as the whole group of parents and children. Of course, since husband and wife are members, they too share in producing this result, however not as husband or wife but as father or mother, as functionaries of the family association.

Family density is considered important because of its impact on family functioning, so that the stronger the family is constituted the greater the protection it offers. The same 'law' is said to apply to political societies, with Durkheim arguing that the suicide rate falls during political upheavals and great wars because society is more strongly integrated and the individual participates more actively in collective life, thereby restricting his egoism and strengthening his will to live.

Just as egoistic suicide is tied to 'excessive individuation' where 'man has become detached from society', altruistic suicide is tied to 'insufficient individuation' where 'social integration is too strong' (Durkheim, 2002: 175). If individuals are bound too tightly to the collective, the argument goes, they value society more than themselves. In contrast to egoistic suicide, which is rooted in 'man's' inability to find a basis for existence in life, altruistic suicide occurs when 'this basis for existence appears to man situated beyond life itself' (2002: 219). In general, Durkheim considers altruistic suicide to be characteristic of 'lower societies', where life is rigorously governed by custom and habit, though it is, he notes, also to be found in modern societies where traditional forms of 'mechanical solidarity' persist such as in the military.

While egoistic and altruistic suicide are attributed to different levels of integration into society, the third of Durkheim's main types of suicide is said to result from 'man's activity lacking regulation and his consequent sufferings' (2002: 219). Anomie, it is argued, is a regular and specific factor in suicide in modern societies, one of the springs from which suicide feeds: hence, by virtue of its origins, this third type is called anomic suicide. When society is disturbed by some painful crisis or abrupt transition, the collective conscience is weakened and society becomes momentarily incapable of regulating individual's desires and their satisfaction. Consequently, a state of normlessness may prevail, upsetting the balance of people's circumstances and broadening their horizons beyond that which they can endure. Anomic suicide is similar to egoistic suicide in that they both 'spring from society's insufficient presence in individuals', but the nature of this absence is different: in egoistic suicide, society is deficient in a 'truly collective activity', whereas in anomic suicide, society's influence is lacking in the 'basically individual passions' leaving them unchecked (2002: 219). Given these differences, Durkheim argued, egoistic and anomic suicide tend to arise in different social environments: namely, intellectual careers or the 'world of thought' and the industrial or commercial world respectively. Industrial and financial crises were said to increase suicide rates, not because of the poverty and hardship they entail, but because the collective order is disturbed and society's regulatory capacity is compromised. So it is that suicide rates were said to increase in times of boom as well as bust.

Another division of anomic suicides is said to result from a weakening of matrimonial regulation due to divorce. The suicidal consequence of divorce were found to be peculiar to men – a pattern that was explained by the suggestion that, for women, marital regulation is a restraint without any great advantages, so that divorce offers a source of protection. While women need liberty, Durkheim argues, men require restraint and widespread, legally sanctioned, divorce weakens the extent to which marriage serves this function: 'in countries where marriage is strongly tempered by divorce', he notes, 'the immunity of the married man is inevitably less. As he resembles the unmarried man under this regime, he inevitably loses some of his own advantages. Consequently, the total number of suicides rises' (2002: 235).

Having delineated the three main types of suicide, Durkheim outlines the individual behaviour-patterns that exemplify them, arguing that the various currents which generate suicide should be followed from their social origins to their individual manifestations. Each victim of suicide, he notes, gives his act 'a personal stamp' which expresses his temperament and particular circumstances, but which cannot be explained by the social and general causes of the phenomenon. Nonetheless, Durkheim insists, these causes 'must stamp the suicides they determine with a shade all their own, a special mark expressive of them' and 'this collective mark we must find' (2002: 241). Noting that the collective mark can only be approximated, he proceeds 'deductively', emphasising the most general and striking characteristics without having an objective criteria for selection. Acts and agents, it is argued, may be classified into a certain number of 'species', which correspond to the main types of suicide and accord with the nature of their social causes, providing 'prolongations of these causes inside of individuals' (2002: 250). The different types of suicide Durkheim identifies are not, by his own admission, always found in a state of purity and isolation, but are very often combined with one another, giving rise to composite or mixed varieties. A 'peculiar' affinity is noted between egoism and anomie, which Durkheim notes, is unsurprising given that these factors are 'usually merely two different aspects of one moral state' (2002: 251).

Whilst recognising that the general characteristics of suicide are complicated by various nuances depending on the personal temperament and specific circumstances of the victim, Durkheim maintains that the immediate antecedents of individual cases are not their determining causes. This is evident, he argues, because these 'individual peculiarities' retain approximately the same relative frequency, while the suicide rate varies considerably. There is, moreover, 'nothing which cannot serve as an occasion for suicide. It all depends on the intensity with which suidogenetic causes have affected the individual' (2002: 264): or, put another way: 'no unhappiness in life necessarily causes a man to kill himself unless he is otherwise so inclined' (2002: 270). The causes of suicide are, therefore, said to be found in the nature of societies themselves for: 'Here at last we are face to face with real laws' (2002: 263):

> The conclusion from all these facts is that the social suicide-rate can be explained only sociologically. At any given moment the moral constitution of society establishes the contingent of voluntary deaths. There is, therefore, for each people a collective force of a definite amount of energy, impelling men to self-destruction. The victim's acts which at first seem to express only his personal temperament are really the supplement and prolongation of a social condition which they express externally.

This collective force, Durkheim explains, is made up of the currents of egoism, altruism and or anomie running through society, which, 'by affecting individuals, cause them to commit suicide' (2002: 264). The private experiences that are usually thought to be the proximate causes of suicide, he insists, only borrow their influence from the victim's moral predisposition, which is, itself, an echo of the moral state of society. As proof of the reality of collective tendencies, Durkheim points to the uniformity of their effects: the regularity of statistical data, he argues, implies the existence of collective tendencies exterior to the individual, which can be directly established in a considerable number of important cases.

Ruth S. Cavan (1965) [1928] *Suicide*

Working under the auspices of the Chicago School, Cavan was one of the first to apply an ecological perspective to suicide. Although Durkheim's work is barely mentioned by Cavan, comparisons between the two studies are instructive. Cavan describes her approach as 'social psychology' and uses a mixed methods approach to develop the central argument that suicide results from social and personal disorganisation. Her book can be regarded as an important early contribution, but strangely Cavan's work is not often cited in contemporary studies of suicide. (Durkheim, however, seems to be a compulsory reference).

Part one of Cavan's study approaches the problem of suicide from the point of view of the group and addresses the questions: 'What phases of social organization develop the tendency to commit suicide, and what phases control and inhibit it or build up alternative types of conduct?' (1965: 11). After a brief historical survey of attitudes to suicide, Cavan turns to contemporary factors, drawing on official statistics, which are said to provide the best basis for comparing suicide rates of different groups, tracing trends, and discovering what factors are associated with suicide. Much of the statistical data is sourced from other writers, including some, such as Morselli, who Durkheim also drew from, though these sources are updated and supplemented with data from the United States. Cavan, like Durkheim before her, uses official statistics to disprove explanations of suicide based on climate and racial temperament, while also drawing attention to differences between religious groups and between urban and rural communities. In so doing, she identifies a range of 'influential determinants' of the suicide rate, including the attitudes and customs of national groups, the breakdown of customs among immigrants, the organising effect and creeds of religious groups and the conditions of urban or rural life.

From here, Cavan goes onto discuss suicide in 'very primitive' and 'very rigid' social organisations or what she also refers to as 'preliterate' and 'oriental' groups. The preliterate situation is said to show the effect of 'simple' homogenous social organisation on personality because: 'There is little disorganization and hence a small amount of personal suicide' (1965: 76). The effects of disorganisation are then examined on the basis of a detailed case study of Chicago, a 'typical American metropolitan center'. For the purposes of statistical and community studies the city was divided into 72 areas and a 'suicide belt' was found to coincide with disorganised communities, including the West Madison area, 'with its womanless street of flophouses, missions, cheap restaurants, and hundreds of men who drift in aimless, bleary-eyed abandon' (1965: 81). Among the activities found to characterise these communities were divorce, 'an indication both of the breakdown of organized family life...and also of the attitude that the family relationship is impermanent' (1965: 93); pawnshops; and murders. Whenever community organisation breaks down, Cavan argues, there is 'an especially good opportunity for personal disorganisation to occur' because 'vagrant and normally inhibited impulses are permitted free reign in a way that is not possible in well-integrated communities' (1965: 104). But community organisation is not considered a direct cause of suicide: 'It is not to be thought that these institutions and types of conduct typical of the highly suicidal areas cause suicide. Rather they are symptoms of a general condition of personal and social disorganization which in the end may lead to suicide' (1965: 104).

Drawing part one to a close, Cavan claims communities which have had stable social organisation are those that have been more or less isolated from contacts with people of diverse customs. A further feature of such societies is said to be almost complete social control, where customs and traditions prescribe behaviour and the needs of the group leave little room for individualism. The small amount of suicide found in such communities is attributed to the lack of individualism and feeling that the individual does not have the right to dispose of life. Conversely, Cavan argues, communities which have had conflicts in social codes and confusion of customs have been those where mobility has aroused new interests and undermined group unity, so that the 'individual stands out as a separate entity, driven by unregulated impulses and wishes and often unable to find satisfaction for them' (1965: 107). In times of social disorganisation, she maintains, many people who would travel happily along under normal circumstances find themselves unable to adjust to confused and conflicting standards, contributing to the increased suicide rates in communities where social disorganisation prevails.

If part one has a largely familiar feel, part two departs from the format laid down by Durkheim by focusing on the individual and examining how personal disorganisation develops and culminates in suicide. According to Cavan the typical situation which causes a European or American to commit suicide is 'intensely personal', it is 'not something which has happened to the group of which he is a member; it is something which has happened to him personally, and the interpretation he places on it is not wholly that of society' (1965: 4). The bulk of this part of the study is based on individual case studies and life histories, which are said to be less exact than statistics, but to provide much more insight into human nature. The personal dimension of suicide is examined through the study of adjustments people try to make when obstacles appear in the on-going process of living – adjustments that are said to be demanded more frequently in an individualistic, changing social order than in a highly socialised, static social order. When adjustments fail 'there may occur a complete breakdown of morale, inability to satisfy fundamental interests, and consequent personal disorganization or demoralization' (1965: 111).

Cavan considers the most marked type of personal disorganisation to be psychosis, but is critical of the tendency to explain suicide in this manner. A large number of people who kill themselves, she notes, are not insane and, even among those who are, suicide is usually precipitated by some crisis, real or imagined. Crises are said to be part of normal living, moreover, and to be multiplied in a changing social order, so that the process of living is, in effect, the process of solving problems or of adjustment. When a 'crucial situation' cannot be resolved in a way that permits the continued pursuit of an 'efficient, normal life' the 'forces of thwarted interests may lead to types of behaviour which are injurious to the person's physical, mental or social welfare and which are usually labelled pathological' (1965: 145). Examples of such behaviour include alcoholism and drug use, sexual perversion, delinquency, insanity and, finally, suicide. Personal disorganisation is then, in Cavan's terms, a lack of adjustment and harmony between the interests that constitute personality and the external world in which life must be lived. While this disorganisation is of several types, she argues, the common theme is that they provide examples of blocking at different stages of what are usually complex acts or enterprises: 'the different types of suicide are really but interruptions which occur at different stages in some definite, ongoing enterprise, whether this be the enterprise of earning money, of securing a wife, or striving for less important things' (1965: 170). When an act is blocked and an alternative plan can not be formulated, there is said to be an accumulation of emotion, which, in the absence of a solution, tends to 'force' some sort of action.

It is these psychological processes, Cavan goes on to argue, that link suicide to the external social world. The social conditions of suicide, she notes, are indicative of the experiences and situations that 'are, at a given time and place, the ones to which it is difficult for people to adjust, and the maladjustment of which leads to discouragement and the feeling that life is intolerable' (1965: 304). These external situations are, nonetheless, only said to be indirectly linked to suicide and to be relevant only insofar as they cause personal disorganisation. In contrast to Durkheim, then, Cavan gives aetiological priority to individual factors, emphasising the role of subjectivity and meaning (1965: 304).

> The essence of the suicidal situation lies in the meaning which it has for the person who experiences it…Disorganization occurs only when the region of life which has become chaotic is regarded as essential and necessary for the person's happiness…The situation is also defined as intolerable, irremediable, hopeless. There is a true psychological crisis. The man who kills himself is through with his life; he has literally died psychologically before he kills his body… It is a crisis which cannot be adjusted to – which ends in defeat. Externally, there may be little or even no evidence of the difficulty, but in his subjective life the person is enduring doubts, unsatisfied longings, and finally hopelessness and inability to struggle longer.

Jack D. Douglas (1967) *The Social Meanings of Suicide*

Douglas sought to lay the foundations for a 'new sociological approach to suicide' or at least one that 'is new in many fundamental respects' (1967: xiv). Drawing on Weber's insights, his approach was based on the claim that suicide should be studied as a form of subjectively meaningful action. A large part of Douglas's case is made up of a critical review of previous studies, starting with Durkheim's contribution, which is said to be the 'cornerstone of the whole approach to suicide taken by almost all sociologists in the twentieth century' (1967: xiii). At the outset, Douglas tells us, his intention was to build on what Durkheim and others had done, but, after encountering some early criticisms of official suicide statistics, he realised he had committed the 'cardinal sin' of not giving careful consideration to his primary source of information. The more he questioned the statistics, Douglas reveals, the more he came to realise they were not what Durkheim and many others had assumed them to be, and the more he analysed Durkheim's study the more convinced he became that it 'was a very complex work' that did not fit the usual interpretations given to it by socio-logists' (1967: viii).

Douglas' review of *Suicide* is critical, yet appreciative. On the plus side, Durkheim was said to have been moving in the direction of studying suicide as meaningful action: hence Douglas' approach was not, by his own admission, 'totally new' (1967: xiv). The predominant positivistic interpretation of *Suicide* is, Douglas claims, a misinterpret-ation, which he attributes to Durkheim's partial ambivalence and to the methodological predilections of contemporary sociologists. Init-ially, Durkheim is said to give the impression of being concerned with the statistical relations between suicide rates and the rates of 'external associations', but: 'If one follows the progress of the work carefully he can see the shift away from the positivistic theory, which made the external social behavior the ultimate cause of suicide, and toward the theory in which the social meanings of behavior are the ultimate determinants of suicide' (1967: 42). With regard to the 'collective rep-resentations' that are most heavily implicated in Durkheim's theory – namely altruism, egoism and anomie – Douglas argues it is 'rather clear' that at least egoism is concerned with *cognitive* meaning and anomie with *affective* meaning. Contrary to Durkheim's claims, more-over, Douglas maintains that these concepts do not refer to sets of morals, so much as to 'orientations toward the (primarily moral) mean-ings that constitute society' (1967: 53). More specifically, he argues, Durkheim's analysis gives the 'clear idea' that the 'integration' of a society is either caused by or defined in terms of shared beliefs, which constitute the ultimate cause(s) of suicide (or, at least, egoistic suicide). Finally, Douglas points to Durkheim's argument that men and women respond to marriage, widowhood, divorce and/or childlessness with different actions because they mean different things to them.

On the down side, *Suicide* is said to bear many of the 'stigmata of ideological warfare' (1967: 73) and its ability to persuade is attributed to the power of its rhetoric rather than integrity of its analysis. Douglas points to several weaknesses in the method, which, he claims, led Durkheim to read meanings into the data to support his theory, including, most notably, a failure to clearly define and explicitly operationalise the main theoretical concepts. Durkheim's residual positivism, it is argued, led him to suppose that individual meanings and interpretations are not theoretically significant and cannot be measured objectively. In the absence of such measures, Durkheim relied upon 'his common-sense understanding of his everyday social experience to provide the most important part of the data to be used to test his theory', while, 'in line with the usual positivistic misunderstanding of statistical data', he generally assumed that 'the data spoke for themselves' (1967: 68). The failure to provide clear definitions, moreover, freed Durkheim to move backwards from the analysis to the meanings of the data and, within loose bounds of common sense, to invoke whatever meanings best fitted his theory. Thus, his work is said to have the 'great fault' of being adjustable in a way that makes it irrefutable. All these problems, Douglas insists, are magnified when we consider that Durkheim knew the 'statistical facts' about suicide and the theoretical ideas used to explain them before he began his study. As such, Douglas concludes, it would be unjustified to believe that Durkheim successfully demonstrated what he thought he had; and yet (1967: 76):

> *Suicide* remains the best sociological work on suicide, primarily because of the *ideal* of scientific investigation of social phenomena which it built on and because in the final analysis it broke with the positivistic tradition of research on suicide, the tradition which was so antithetical to the treatment of suicide as actions caused by social meanings.

The 'post-Durkheimian' sociological theories of suicide are, according to Douglas, relatively superficial and fragmentary. Most, he notes, are influenced by Durkheim's work and, therefore, share some obvious similarities and redundancies. Even the ecological perspectives such as Cavan's, which was developed outside the Durkheimian tradition, were greatly influenced by Morselli, so that they too shared fundamental elements with Durkheim's analysis. Foremost among the general problems noted by Douglas, many of these studies were said to have adopted a 'causistic-deductive' method, yet try to give the impression they have used a deductive method, whereby they move from the data to the theory: 'This positivistic rhetoric', he notes, 'has often given a scientific aura to these works when the actual methods used were anything but scientific' (1967: 153). Uncritical treatment of the data is identified as a common problem, with official records being assumed to offer valid and reliable data that will unlock the secrets of social action. It is also noted that implicitly, at least, many studies assume individual or immediate causes of specific suicides to be too complex to be included in any systematic theory. Consequently, the meaning of suicide and associated social norms are generally taken for granted and assumed to be both culturally homogenous and readily accessible to the sociological observer. Ecological perspectives, are, once again, considered something of an exception. According to Douglas, the likes of Cavan downplayed the ecological aspects of their work in an attempt to avoid the ecological fallacy and, in so doing, placed greater emphasis on the importance of social and individual meanings to suicide, albeit without developing these ideas systematically.

As well as rejecting the theoretical orientation of most previous studies, Douglas criticises their reliance on official statistics. The 'fundamental weakness' of all but a few of these studies, he argues, is that the data are inadequate for their theoretical purposes: that is, official statistics are assumed to represent one thing when they actually represent many things or, rather, are the product of many complicated social processes. Differing definitions and search procedures, Douglas argues, render official suicide statistics 'invalid' and 'incomparable'. Concealment is also identified as a potential source of systematic bias, which has significant implications for established theories. Catholics, it is argued, tend to condemn suicide much more severely than Protestants or Jews, with the result that they attempt to hide it much more and, as a general proposition: 'We would then expect that *the more socially integrated an individual is, the more he and his significant others will try to avoid having his death categorised as a suicide*' (1967: 209, original emphasis). The main error in the use of official statistics, Douglas concludes, is the same as that contained in the theories themselves: 'that is the assumption that "suicidal actions" have a necessary and sufficient, unidimensional meaning' (1967: 229). This error, he argues, is a function of the basic weakness of the 'statistical-hypothetical' or 'positivistic' approach: namely, the failure to 'take into consideration the fact that *social meanings are fundamentally problematic, both for the members of society and for the scientists attempting to observe, describe and explain their actions*' (1967: 339, original emphasis).

Douglas' critique of previous studies and the 'statistical-hypothetical' approach leads to the central assumption underlying his preferred alternative: 'namely, that we should begin *as far as is possible* with a study of the real world phenomena, above all with a study of the meanings of these phenomena to the social participants' (1976: 82, original emphasis). What is considered important here is the 'inside story' or the 'subjective meanings' to the social actors involved and this requires that attention be given to the statements and actions of people in everyday life. The meanings of suicidal phenomena within Western culture, Douglas argues, are highly ambiguous, so that the specific, actualised meanings of these phenomena have to be constructed by the individuals involved based on shared cultural meanings and the shared context of meanings given to them by their past interactions. Gaining insight into such processes requires information that 'deals with individuals as individuals' (1976: 255) and Douglas draws mainly on 'psychiatric case studies' augmented by 'artistic sources' and, 'perhaps most importantly, the uninformed and informed experience with suicidal phenomena of the theorist in everyday life' (1976: 264). Suicidal actions, he notes, are generally taken to mean something is fundamentally wrong with the situation of the actor at the time and it is this 'reflexive dimension' that makes suicidal actions effective social weapons. Suicidal actions are also taken to mean something fundamental about the actor 'himself', so that, when properly performed, they can be used to transform the substantial self. From here, Douglas goes onto identify 'those patterns of actions and meanings which seem, from a general survey of the literature in the Western world on suicide, to be most frequent' and 'are very likely those...which are distinctive of suicidal actions' (1976: 284). Among these fundamental meanings, suicidal actions are said to offer a way of transforming the soul from this world to the other world, which is often construed as a form of 'escape'; of transforming the substantial self in this world or the other world; of achieving fellow feeling; and of getting revenge. Ultimately, however, Douglas concludes that the 'serious shortage of good descriptions has prevented us from advancing very far toward our general goal of explaining suicidal actions as meaningful actions' (1967: 340). Nonetheless, he maintains, the immediate goal before us must be that of providing careful, comparative descriptions of social action for it is only when this has been done that we can get on with the general task of constructing more abstract theories to explain social action.

J. Maxwell Atkinson (1978) *Discovering Suicide: Studies in the Social Organization of Sudden Death*

Atkinson also makes the case for a constructionist approach to the study of suicide. Although partially motivated by an interest in the nature and validity of official data, his original intention was not to 'disprove' or 'invalidate' Durkheim's theories, but to find a way of calculating 'more accurate' suicide rates so as to better assess them. From this 'naively "positivist"' (1978: 4) starting point, Atkinson went on to develop a distinctly critical perspective. Sociology's relationship with suicide, he argues, is a paradoxical one that can best be characterised as 'fascination from a distance' (1978: 9). Bemoaning the lack of empirical engagement, suicide was said to have provided a convenient vehicle for broader sociological concerns: 'it was the *issues* posed by Durkheim in a book which just happened to be on suicide, rather than the *phenomenon of suicide* itself which has stimulated most of the sociological interest' (1978: 31). For all that theorists, methodologists and text book writers have to say on the subject, sociology was deemed to be of little help to the would-be researcher when faced 'with fundamental and unsolved methodological problems which appear so obvious that it initially seems strange that they have been given so little attention in the past' (1978: 31).

Atkinson's own research followed a 'somewhat turbulent course', shifting from 'positivism to interactionism to ethnomethodology' (1978: 6). These changes were partly driven by his attempts to explore theoretical ideas in empirical settings, prompting the claim that 'obsessive empiricism can point to the need for a paradigm shift by generating findings which can not be made sense of in any other way' (1978: 7). The transition to interactionism was facilitated by contact with the sociology of deviance and came 'fairly easily' because it fitted with Atkinson's pre-existing concerns about official statistics as well as his interest in labelling and societal reaction. Quite what was involved in the departure from positivism began to be specified in his review of suicide research and data derived from official sources. In keeping with the main tenets of interactionism, Atkinson charts a growing concern over the problems of using such data, while criticising the way in which these problems were being conceived in a way that was consistent with the Durkheimian tradition. Suicides, he complained, are almost universally assumed to be relatively clearly defined events, so that the problem is considered to be a technical one of reliability and validity, with little consideration of broader issues: 'Asking questions about the appropriateness of that way of doing science is in no way a part of the scientific enterprise which has come to be known as "suicidology"' (1978: 61). With the exception of Douglas, Atkinson claims, suicide researchers appear unaware or unconcerned with any alternative formulations, describing their responses to the problems that had been identified as inadequate and unscientific. There is ultimately, he notes, 'still no evidence which warrants the conclusion that analyses based on officially derived data can be continued as if there were no significant problem' (1978: 66).

Drawing inspiration from the interactionist approach to deviance and Douglas' work on suicide, Atkinson attempts to develop a model of the suicide process as a guide for empirical research. Various research strategies were tried but a series of practical and theoretical problems emerged which, he argues, raised doubts about Douglas' analysis and the various interactionist approaches to deviance. Operationalising the 'sequential' model of deviance favoured by interactionists, for example, meant, at some stage, accepting other people's definitions of suicide at face value. Douglas' work, moreover, 'seems to diminish in clarity at the very point when his "new approach" to the sociology of suicide was to have been articulated and demonstrated in action' (1978: 79). 'Vagueness' and 'mistakes' meant 'no clear directives' are provided as to 'how new empirical work should be done or in what form it should take' (1978: 83). As a further complication, it was said to be unclear from the interactionist or other sociological literature what one should do next in light of the kinds of findings that were being produced.

The rest of the research that Atkinson reports was carried out 'in an attempt to find ways of studying what seemed to be among the most important of the problems Douglas poses' (1978: 83). Initial inquiries uncovered significant difficulties in locating what seemed to be the least problematic of the different types of definition: namely an official legal one. Despite these difficulties (1978: 108–9):

> ...it appeared from our evidence that it was possible for a coroner to be unable to provide an approximation to the official definition of suicide...and yet to be able routinely to generate official cate-gorizations without arousing any criticism or doubts about his competence. The implication of this is that the procedures for cate-gorizing sudden deaths are organized in some *unknown* way which cannot be anticipated in advance of research.

Thus formulated, Atkinson's research question became, how do deaths get characterised as suicides?, and this led to detailed consid-eration of the processes by which such verdicts are recorded. When faced with a case of sudden death, the 'abiding concern' of coroners' officers is to 'achieve order out of chaos' (1978: 172). Given the legal need to establish intent, this means more than simply establishing the cause of death and requires that a motive or plausible explanation be provided as to why the deceased should have taken their own life. Coroners arrive at such explanations, Atkinson argues, by apply-ing 'common sense' theories based on 'taken-for-granted' assumptions about what constitutes a 'typical suicide', a 'typical suicidal bio-graphy' and so on. Rather than treating 'suicide notes', 'modes of dying', 'circumstances of death' and 'biographical factors' as sep-arate or independent items, moreover, coroners are said to develop composites, so that features of a particular death may only come to be viewed as indicative of suicide in light of biographical data that are regarded as indicative of a possible suicide or vice versa. Coroners, it is noted, have ideas about which modes of dying are typically suicidal as well as the kinds of circumstances that lead people to commit suicide and use these ideas, together with certain 'cues', to build an explanatory model of how each death occurred. For a suicide verdict to be recorded, Atkinson concludes, no part of the model must be inconsistent with the coroner's ideas about factors that are typically associated with suicide. The importance 'of this prac-tice for the social organization of sudden death is that it provides for the construction of a plausible story of how and why the death

occurred without which uncertainty and disorder would prevail'
(1978: 172).

   Coroners are not alone in constructing such stories and the involvement of relatives, witnesses, journalists and the like is deemed
highly significant. Arguing that 'lay' explanations rely on very similar,
albeit less sophisticated, processes to those used by officials, Atkinson
suggests that there are tautological forces at work here. The cues that
coroners use as indicators of intent are said to bear a very close resem-
blance to the variables experts use to explain suicide, so that *'all
or most of the "causes" cited by suicidologists are indeed "involved" in the
very description of suicide'* (1978: 172, original emphasis). By extension
(1978: 143):

> The implications of this kind of analysis for suicide research
> which depends on the correlational work with data derived from
> coroners' records are clearly very serious. By showing relation-
> ships between variables like marital status, mental illness, alco-
> holism, economic disaster and so on with suicide, it is arguable
> that all the researchers are doing is to make explicit the explana-
> tions used implicitly by coroners in their everyday work.

Atkinson's final chapter is given over to ethnomethodology, which,
he proposes, 'promises an answer, and possibly the only answer to
the problems' that remain (1967: 187). Given the controversies and
misunderstandings surrounding this approach, Atkinson provides
a general assessment of ethnomethodology and its (possible) applications to suicide, though, by his own admission, he would have
preferred to present some preliminary attempts at an ethnomethodological analysis of empirical materials. Ethnomethodology, it is noted,
is centrally concerned with the intersubjective character of social reality
and implies a rejection of rival forms of analyses. What other sociological perspectives typically treat as a resource, ethnomethodology
treats as a *topic*, focusing on the methods members use to make sense
of the social world and achieve coherence or social order. Viewed thus,
the main problem with Durkheim's *Suicide* is not the reliance on official statistics but the assumption that events occur which sociologists
should consider 'really suicide'. All utterances and actions, it is argued,
are indexical, in the sense that their meaning depends on the context,
so what really needs to be considered is the way members routinely

'repair' or resolve inherent ambiguity. Applied to suicide this means investigating how a decision that a suicide has occurred is reached and how an object must be conceived in order to talk of it as 'committing' suicide.

According to ethnomethodologists the everyday problems of indexicality are akin to the problems faced by sociologists, while members' methods are said to involve 'practical sociological reasoning'. These parallels, Atkinson notes, help to explain the similarities between lay and official explanations of sudden death. The focus on members' methods also distinguishes ethnomethodology from other sociological work that is concerned with meaning, including that of Douglas and the interactionists: 'Ethnomethodologists are not interested in the endless elaboration of indexical particulars or in the simple reportage of repairs that members do, but are concerned with the discovery of members' methods for repairing indexical particulars' (1978: 183). The breakthrough here, insists Atkinson, is that ethnomethodology takes the problem of *how* members' categorisations are accomplished as a central and fundamental problem in studying social order and shows how such a task may be started. The irony, though, is that when such an approach is taken sudden deaths lose their distinctiveness because it is the situated methods themselves that become the prime concern rather than the particular categorisation being selected: and 'deaths get categorized as suicides in much the same way as anything else gets categorized' (1978: 196). Ultimately then, as far as the continued study of suicide as a topic is concerned, 'ethnomethodology has no glib or easy solution' (1978: 197).

The king is dead, long live the king

Sociology remains a bit-part player in contemporary suicide studies. It was noted in the Introduction that a search of the Institute for Scientific Information (ISI) in 2009 by Agerbo *et al.* (2009) found that of more than 30,000 academic papers published on the subject since 1980 no more than 400 could be categorised as sociological. Despite the best efforts of Douglas and Atkinson, moreover, the vast majority of these papers have continued along well-established lines and broadly Durkheimian in approach. Suicide studies have remained largely impervious to the 'new' approaches advocated by these authors and their programmes of research have remained largely undeveloped. Some sense of why this may be can be gleaned from an early review of Douglas' work in the *Journal of the American Medical Association* (Friedman, 1968: 232):

> Prolixity, complexity and semantic haggling characterize the author's style....Douglas seems reluctant to accept the simple, the common-sensical. This presentation may have some appeal to sociologists and psychologists. Busy physicians – pragmatic and practical, devoted to the task of saving lives – can spare little time for this sort of arm-chair philosophizing and semantic juggling.

To the extent that Douglas and Atkinson have had a lasting impact on suicide studies they have done so by reawakening interest in the accuracy of official statistics (Lindqvist and Gustafsson, 2002; Pesco-solido and Mendelsohn, 1986; Platt *et al.*, 1988), with some, albeit fairly peripheral, on-going interest in their substantive concerns (see, for example, Timmermans, 2005; Whitt, 2006). Although the problem of reliability 'simply haunts suicide research' (Gibbs, 1994: 62), the challenge posed by Douglas, in particular, was followed by a reassertion of the value and utility of official statistics. For some, such confidence was grounded in carefully constructed evidence, though 'most efforts targeting the etiology of suicide fail to address the criticisms that have plagued the empirical study of suicide and continue to take for granted the use of official aggregate data on suicide' (Pescosolido, 1994: 269).

The most influential sociological perspective on suicide remains that developed by Durkheim, the legacy of which continues to be felt both within and beyond sociology. That Durkheim's place as the chief 'paradigm innovator' remains undisturbed is evident from the collected works that were produced to mark the centenary of the publication of *Suicide* (Lester, 1994; Pickering and Walford, 2000): 'At base, the Durkheimian framework remains the standard, it has characteristics that make it both elegant and powerful' (Pescosolido, 1994: 291) and 'there is good evidence that Durkheim's theory of ego-istic suicide is correct and that it can be extended' (Breault, 1994: 24). Although less celebrated outside of sociology, the value of Durkheim's work continues to be recognised, albeit grudgingly at times. A recent review of *Suicide* in an international psychiatric journal insisted that

Durkheim's scientific method and argument are 'fundamentally flawed' and his thesis is significantly limited by the 'baseless' dismissal of mental illness as a key determinant of suicidal behaviour, but went on to note that some of his concepts have 'instrumental value': in particular, it noted that the conceptualisation of anomic, egoistic and altruistic suicide 'provides a means of comprehending recent trends in suicidal behaviour in the former Soviet states and a possible window into the psyche of the suicides of religious and political extremists' (Robertson, 2006: 365).

Reflecting Durkheim's legacy, suicide studies remain relentlessly quantitative in their methods, with less than 3 per cent of articles published in the three international suicide research journals between 2005 and 2007 being based on qualitative research (Hjelmeland and Knizek, 2010). The complexity of Durkheim's work has led many researchers to focus on particular testable elements of the theory, often by comparing suicide rates between groups or societies (Pescosolido, 1994). Such studies have confirmed certain elements of Durkheim's analysis: in almost every country where records are kept, for example, men kill themselves in far greater numbers than women (Baudelot and Establet, 2008; but see Kushner, 1994); marriage has generally been found to be a protective factor and divorce an aggravating factor (Stack, 2000b); while a recently completed 'two-hundred-year-long world tour' supported the conclusion that suicide 'rates always rise during economic crises, and fall during wars' (Baudelot and Establet, 2008: 179). Some of Durkheim's other claims have been less well supported. The 'near obsession with religion and suicide' has uncovered numerous populations where the pattern described in *Suicide* does not hold (Gibbs, 1994: 66) and research on modernisation, religious integration and political integration has often questioned or reformulated the traditional Durkheimian perspective (Stack, 2000b). Durkheim's propositions on the economy and suicide have been found to be 'largely wrong' and his claims about an inverse relationship have been refuted: far from increasing suicide, prosperity and high socio-economic standing decrease it, so that lower-income groups have a higher suicide rate than higher income groups (Stack, 1994: 246; 2000b). While the effect of war on suicide has been found to be spurious (Stack, 2000b), moreover, Durkheim appears to have been too ready to dismiss the influence of imitation and alcoholism: recent research has identified a 'copy cat' effect associated with the mass media in the United States, Germany and Japan and has also demonstrated a clear link between alcohol consumption and suicide across many different jurisdictions (Stack, 2000a).

As well as guiding empirical endeavours, Durkheim's legacy can be seen in recent theoretical developments. Status integration theory, for example, was inspired by Durkheim, whose influence is clearly evident in the theory's first postulate: that the suicide rate of a population varies inversely with the stability and durability of social relationships within that population (Gibbs, 1994). Similarly, Pescosolido's social network approach, which focuses on the role that social ties play in creating social structures and providing a mechanism through which they influence attitudes, beliefs and behaviours, is also 'consistent with the central thrust of Durkheim's work and its application to "postmodern" society' (1994: 266).

Although dominant, Durkheim's influence is not absolute and there are signs that the prevailing paradigm might be fragmenting. According to one of the leading academics in the field, historical trends, including a long-term decline in the suicide rate in some countries and a levelling off in others, 'warrant a rethinking of many of Durkheim's basic axioms' (Stack, 1994: 246). Calls for more qualitative research (Hjelmeland and Knizek, 2010), moreover, have been matched by growing interest in studying individual cases, rather than rates, of suicide (Maris, 1981; see Gibbs, 1994; Stack and Wasserman, 2007). At the same time, innovative theoretical perspectives have linked suicide and suicide risk to musical subcultures, alcohol consumption, economic strain due to relative cohort size and opportunity factors such as gun availability and the use of toxic gas in domestic appliances (Stack, 2000a). Without Durkheim there may well have been no sociology of suicide, but, as some have noted, his legacy is jeopardised more by veneration than by anti-positivist criticisms: 'Hence, sociologists should rightly proclaim Durkheim to have been a genius, *and then get on with it*' (Gibbs, 1994: 30, original emphasis).

Getting on with it, but how?

The sociology of suicide has been shaped by a series of divisions and oppositions, with most commentators retreating into schools of thought that perpetuate the polarised nature of debate (Taylor, 1994). There are, as a result, several related, yet distinct, questions which any sociology of suicide should seek to address: can suicide be thought of as social fact or is it a social construct with little external validity? Is suicide best understood as a collective or individual phenomenon? What methods are best used to study suicide? What is distinct about a sociological approach to suicide and what is its relationship with psychology? The broader issues underlying these questions are, of course, not unique to the study of suicide and nor are the answers. Sociology as a whole has been similarly beset by a series of unhelpful dichotomies, including those drawn between subjectivism and objectivism, social structure and human agency, quantitative and qualitative methods, and it is to the parent discipline that we must turn for something like a solution. Many, if not all, of these dichotomies have been challenged in some way or another (see Jenks, 1998; Bryman, 2004) and the contributions of Anthony Giddens and Pierre Bourdieu are particularly significant in this regard.

In *New Rules of Sociological Method*, Giddens (1976) argues that social science should 'move out of the shadow of natural science, in whatever philosophical mantle the latter may be clad' (1976: 14), insisting that its subject matter is fundamentally different in that it deals with a universe that has already been rendered meaningful by social actors themselves. While emphasising the role of subjectivity, Giddens criticises interpretive perspectives for their preoccupation with meaning; their tendency to explain all human conduct in terms of motives at the expense of causal conditions; and their failure to relate social norms to asymmetries of power and social divisions. The relationship between human agency and social structure is considered in some detail with a view to clearing up some of the epistemological difficulties that are said to limit the logic of social scientific method. While rejecting the determinism of structural perspectives, Giddens acknowledges the bounded nature of human agency: '*Men produce society, but they do so as historically located actors, and not under conditions of their own choosing*' (1976: 160, original emphasis). While society, he notes, is produced through the skilled performance of its members, this performance draws upon resources, and depends on conditions, which they may be unaware of, or perceive, only dimly. Thus, social structures are said to be constituted by human agency, yet simultaneously provide the medium through which society is constituted. Accordingly, structures should be examined in terms of their 'structuration', that is, as a series of reproduced practices (see also Giddens,

1984). A key methodological point that flows from this analysis is as follows: if agency and structure are not easily separable, then it is neither necessary nor desirable to have separate epistemologies to study them.

Bourdieu offers a similar set of propositions, but is much more explicit about the implications they have for the immediate practice of social research (Bourdieu and Wacquant, 1992; Jenkins, 1992). As well as challenging the division between subjectivism and objectivism, Bourdieu emphasises the interplay between social structure and human agency, prompting some commentators to describe him as a proponent of structuration (Jenkins, 1992; but see Wacquant, 1992). Social divisions, Bourdieu argues, are embodied in mental schemata and the correspondence between these dimensions is reflected in the peculiar 'double life' of social structures. While existing as material phenomena in the 'objectivity of the first order', these structures also exist as symbolic templates for practical activities in the 'objectivity of the second order'. The aim of sociology, then, is to uncover both social structures and the mechanisms by which they are reproduced or transformed. To this end, Bourdieu advocates a social praxeology, whereby structural and phenomenological approaches are integrated into an epistemologically coherent mode of inquiry. Accordingly, mundane representations are initially pushed aside in order to construct the objective structures whose articulations can be materially observed, measured and mapped out independently of the representations of those who live in them. Using statistics, ethnography or formal modelling, the external observer can decode the 'unwritten musical score according to which the actions of agents, each of whom believes she is improvising their own melody, are organized' (Bourdieu, 1980: 89). The immediate, lived experience of agents is then reintroduced in order to explicate the categories of perception and appreciation that structure their actions. While Bourdieu grants epistemological priority to the objectivist reading, the correspondence between mental and social structures means that 'analysis of objective structures logically carries over into the analysis of subjective dispositions' (Bourdieu and de Saint Martin, 1982: 47).

The social world, Bourdieu notes, does not follow the neat regularity of a normative or judicial principle, so that the 'peculiar difficulty of sociology...is to produce a precise science of an imprecise, fuzzy, woolly reality' (Wacquant, 1992: 23). It follows, therefore, that the ambiguities involved in suicide do not necessarily preclude the possibility of systematic study, though they undoubtedly present difficulties of definition and measurement. As a working definition, suicide may be said to occur when somebody wilfully takes their own life, but there are some grey areas involved here. If somebody is admitted to hospital having taken an overdose and dies from a secondary infection, or if somebody jumps to their death from a building under the delusional belief they can fly, can they be said to have committed suicide? Questions of intent also pose significant difficulties of measurement and raise significant doubts about the validity of official suicide records. Because it cannot be observed directly, intent must be inferred on the basis of witness reports, suicide notes, suicide guidelines, previous attempts, testimonials, life crises and mode of death (Timmermans, 2005; see also Lindqvist and Gustafsson, 2002). Officials tend to be fairly conservative when making such inferences, moreover, with the result that suicides are generally undercounted, albeit to a degree that varies across time and space (Whitt, 2006).

Despite the problems of definition and measurement, suicide records are less seriously compromised than is sometimes suggested. Several commentators have noted that Douglas (1967) asserted, rather than demonstrated, flaws in official statistics and subsequent analyses have encouraged a consensus that official statistics can be used, albeit with caution, to assess the causes of suicidal behaviour (Whitt, 2006; see also Gibbs, 1994. Early research by Sainsbury and Barraclough (1968) found suicide rates among immigrant populations in the United States to be very strongly correlated with rates in their country of origin and, drawing on data from England and Wales, also indicated that changes of personnel (coroners in this case) have a negligible effect on the suicide rate. Further research suggests that the number of equivocal cases is small (O'Carroll, 1989); that combining suicides with accidental and undetermined deaths does not appreciably alter research findings (Sainsbury and Jenkins, 1982); and that the social construction of suicide does not invalidate official records because misreporting 'has little discernable impact on the effects of variables commonly used to test sociological theories of suicide' (Pescosolido and Mendelsohn, 1986: 80; see also Platt *et al.*, 1988).

Given that official suicide statistics retain some validity, it is difficult to disagree with Giddens' judgment that *Suicide* 'represents a brilliant vindication of Durkheim's fundamental thesis that social facts can be studied as "realities external to the individual"' (1965: 10); or, more recently, that 'the study remains a classic and his fundamental assertion remains: even the seemingly personal act of suicide demands a sociological explanation' (Giddens, 2006: 15). In view of this endorsement, it is important to note that Durkheim was not the arch positivist he is often assumed to be and was neither indifferent to the role of meaning nor opposed to the study of the individual. His opposition was to individualistic perspectives in which individual consciousness is accepted as an explanation for people's actions (Taylor, 1994). Nonetheless, some of the theoretical problems Durkheim posed were 'pseudo-problems' – that is, problems falsely posed (Gurvitch, 1939) and the dichotomy he drew between the individual and society is one such problem (Giddens, 1965). Additionally, Durkheim's preoccupation with suicide rates entails some notable silences and leaves important questions unanswered: his analysis does not explain why some members of a social group kill themselves while others do not, nor why people kill themselves when they do – the claims he makes in this regard are, as we shall see in Chapter 7, among the least satisfactory aspects of his analysis. Although aggregate analysis of rates may provide reliable predictors of individual behaviour under some circumstances (Breault, 1994), elements of the ecological fallacy remain. As Douglas (1967: 158) notes: 'To explain an exceedingly small number of suicides in terms of the external properties which these individuals have in common with huge numbers of individuals in the same society is to argue in a manner that must surely be given the most critical scrutiny'. Subjective dimensions remain important, for all the reasons outlined by Cavan (1965 [1928]) and Douglas (1967).

Suicide, then, may be said to have a peculiar double life, existing as structured practice in the 'objectivity of the first order' (albeit in a fuzzy and vague way) and embodied in the corresponding mental schemata that provide symbolic templates for practical activities in the 'objectivity of the second order'. To inquire into suicide, therefore, is to inquire into the interplay between these related forms of existence and, as such, suicide might be usefully thought of as a reproduced practice. Under the influence of certain social norms and subjective meanings, an individual may come to consider suicide a viable response to a set of conditions that are, almost by definition, not (entirely) of their own making. By taking their own life, the individual, in turn, reinforces the norms and subjective meanings that define suicide as a viable response to such conditions.

What then of the relationship between sociology and psychology? Of all the divisions that are evident in suicidology that between sociology and psychology is, perhaps, the most perplexing, not least because it is more apparent than real. Almost all the studies that have considered suicide to be a fundamentally social phenomenon actually offer 'psycho-social theories' (Douglas, 1967: 152). Not even Durkheim (2002: 276) completely rejected psychology, noting, in one of his more conciliatory moments:

> But by separating social from individual life in this manner, we do not mean that there is nothing psychical about the former. On the contrary, it is clear that essentially social life is made up of representations. Only these collective representations are of quite another character from those of the individual. We see no objection to calling sociology a variety of psychology, if we carefully add that social psychology has its own laws which are not those of individual psychology.

So it is that Durkheim's work has been described as a 'general social psychological theory' of suicide with an affinity to Freudian psychoanalysis (Taylor, 1994: 7; see Simpson, 1951; Stack, 1994). While several subsequent attempts have been made to integrate sociological and psychological explanations (see Blondel, 1933; Henry and Short, 1954; Gold, 1958), nowhere is this affinity more clearly evident than in Giddens' (1971) exploration of the psychoanalytic dimensions of egoistic and anomic suicide. The factors governing the distribution of the suicide in a community cannot, Giddens (1965) contends, be usefully considered in isolation from those determining why one person commits suicide while another does not. Durkheim's analysis, he notes, is complicated and sometimes ambiguous, with the result that sociologists tend to regard anomic and egoistic suicide as indistinguishable from one another. Whilst recognising the impossibility of drawing an absolute line between them, Giddens (1971) maintains that it is not difficult to separate egoism from anomie as general conditions of social structure. Consequently, he sought to conceptualise the distinction between egoistic and anomic suicide in a way that is clear, internally coherent and consistent with research evidence.

Put simply, egoism relates to social integration, while anomie relates to normative integration. Egoism tends towards the isolation of individuals from closely defined ties with others, so that egoistic suicide is 'an attempt to influence others through self-punishment, and thereby to escape from social isolation' (1971: 113). Anomie, on the other hand, embraces most spheres of social activity or situations where 'failure' is possible, with social and psychological factors coming together to 'push' the individual towards detachment from defined and realisable goals. If life seems meaningless, under such conditions, it is not because of separation from others, but because activities are not structured by aspirations which accord with the identity a person has achieved. Actual cases of suicide, Giddens confirms, may involve both egoistic and anomic currents and must be judged according to how far they tend towards one or the other. On a more general note, his emphasis on the confluence between psychological and sociological factors provides a recurring theme in our analysis.

Conclusion

The studies of suicide we have featured in this chapter are thoroughly permeated by the grand themes of sociology. Spanning most of the last century, the work of Durkheim (2002 [1897]), Cavan (1965 [1928]), Douglas (1967) and Atkinson (1978) pivot on a series of core sociological dichotomies and oppositions. These separations, we have argued, are, in many respects, more apparent than real, resting on artificial divisions and posing 'pseudo problems'.

Drawing inspiration from the work of Giddens and Bourdieu, we have begun to sketch out a way in which we might move beyond these oppositions to develop a more rounded view of suicide. Ours is an inclusive approach that is sympathetic to interpretive sociology, but does not abandon the hope of a generalising social science which is sensitive to meaning whilst simultaneously being concerned with underlying causal processes. The details of our approach will be fleshed out in the coming pages, but the basic idea is that the double life of suicide requires a double reading. To this end, we have taken what we term a 'dual paradigms' approach, which respects both constructionism and objectivism. In the light of Atkinson's work, it seems impossible to ignore the way that knowledge about suicide is constructed and this provides the starting point of our empirical analysis. Chapters 4 and 5 provide a constructionist reading of coroner's inquests and suicide notes respectively, with a view to identifying some of the social processes involved and assessing what they tell us about the wider social and cultural context within which suicidal acts should be understood. Thereafter our focus shifts on to the lived experiences of suicidal individuals and the circumstances in which they take their own life (insofar as they can be recovered). The analysis culminates in Chapter 7 with a largely quantitative reading of our 100 cases and seeks to show how suicidal behaviour is structured by broader social relations. By providing a double reading we hope to capture the structural dimensions of suicide while remaining sensitive to the meanings and motivations of the individuals involved.

3
What is a Sociological Autopsy?

The dichotomies and oppositions that permeate the sociology of suicide have given rise to very different research strategies, though quantitative approaches in the Durkheimian tradition remain dominant. Our emphasis on the need to transcend artificial divisions in understanding, whether they be based on agency and structure, the individual and the social, psychology and sociology, carries over into the methodological realm. The central problem here was neatly encapsulated by Kay Redfield Jamison (2000: 20), professor of psychiatry at Johns Hopkins University and herself a survivor of suicide attempts, when she wrote:

> It should not be necessary, at the end of a century so rich in literature, medicine, psychology, and science, to draw arbitrary lines in the sand between humanism and individual complexities, on the one hand, and clinical or scientific understandings, on the other. That they are bound and beholden to each other should be obvious. Yet it is undeniable that Maginot Lines exist.

Although Jamison's comments are not limited to *social* science, they highlight the disciplinary and methodological divide between approaches that focus on the complex stories of individuals and those that seek to develop scientifically robust generalisations. The Maginot Lines she mentions are, of course, very familiar within sociology and reflect the kind of divisions we drew attention to earlier. Our intention in this chapter is to cross at least one of the Maginot lines Jamison refers to by arguing for a method which uses case-based and variable-based analysis in an attempt to encompass both reasonably objective evidence about the social contexts of individual suicides and a constructionist emphasis on how knowledge about these suicides is produced. We start by outlining the basis of the quantitative/qualitative divide, before going onto to examine the case for combining these types of method. We then discuss our preferred strategy, explaining what we mean by a dual paradigm approach and sociological autopsy. This strategy rests on a qualitatively-led mixed methods approach (Mason, 2006) that is, we hope, consistent with C. Wright Mills' (1959) call for a creative, lateral-thinking, problem-oriented social science.

Paradigm wars

The strength of the quantitative/qualitative divide can be gauged from the way in which it tends to be characterised using military metaphors. Advocates of each type of approach are said to form 'armed camps' (see Silverman, 2001) and the exchanges between them are routinely described as 'paradigm wars' (see Oakley, 1999). Although debates about quantitative and qualitative research can be traced back to the mid-nineteenth century (Hammersley, 1992), the 'battle' between them only really came to prominence during the 1950s and 1960s, when advocates of the interpretative paradigm attacked the positivistic inclinations of mainstream sociology.

The challenge that interpretivism posed to positivism was spelled out most clearly by Herbert Blumer (1956, 1969), who was principally concerned with the epistemological implications of symbolic interactionism. Blumer's critique centred on the limitations of what he disparagingly referred to as 'scientism' and 'variable analysis'. Because sociological notions are typically abstract and lack any fixed or uniform indicators, he argued, any claim to be able to measure them is spurious. According to Blumer, social science variables are not clear and discrete 'objects' with precisely defined properties and are nothing more than 'abbreviated terms of reference' for complex patterns of social organisation. Except in the most basic of ways, therefore, they do not express quantifiable relations between known dimensions. Blumer also criticised variable analysis for drawing on a faulty stimulus-response model of social interaction, which views human action as a relatively automatic response to external stimuli. In opposing this model, he emphasised the deliberative and creative

nature of human action, arguing that the meaning of social circumstances depends on the plans, purposes and knowledge of the social
actor. Accordingly, the process of interpretation through which
actors construct their actions was considered to provide the appropriate focus for social research and a 'naturalistic' approach based on
detailed studies of particular situations and settings was favoured. The
starting point for such an approach was not provided by abstract concepts, moreover, but by a desire to learn, at first hand, about the way
such situations are experienced by those involved in them. In practice,
this commonly translated into preference for qualitative methods,
particularly ethnography and depth interviews.

Blumer's critique proved highly influential and paved the way for
the flourishing of interpretive sociology during the 1960s. Another
highly significant driving force behind the 'paradigm war' that followed was provided by the arrival of feminism as a political and
social movement. Feminists, notes Oakley, 'underscored the importance for political reasons of using "qualitative" research methods,
and gave an altogether new gloss to anti-science critiques of quantification' (1999: 248). In time, then, Blumer's critique gave rise to
a general consensus that quantitative and qualitative methods represent separate research paradigms which are rooted in different, and
arguably incompatible, ontological and epistemological commitments
(Bryman, 2004). Thus, for example, quantitative research came to be
characterised as a research strategy that not only emphasises quantification, but also embraces a hypothetico-deductive approach that is
sympathetic to the natural scientific model and views the social world
as an external, objective reality. Qualitative research, by contrast, came
to be characterised as a research strategy that focuses on words rather
than numbers, favours an inductive approach, rejects the natural
scientific model, and views the world around us as a social construct
that is in a constant state of (re)negotiation.

The construction of a separate qualitative 'paradigm' significantly
altered the sociological landscape. To extend the military metaphor,
the once besieged qualitative 'camp' fought its way out of the trenches
and mounted a successful counter-attack, of which Douglas (1967)
and Atkinson (1978) were a part. In Britain, at least, methodological
fashion has swung decisively towards qualitative methods (Hammersley, 1992) and quantitative approaches have come to be viewed with
considerable suspicion and scepticism: 'Since the 1960s', notes David

Silverman 'a story has got about that no good sociologists should dirty their hands with numbers' (2001: 35). The decline of quantitative research has been noted with alarm in some quarters and has been confirmed by a recent review of mainstream British journals which found that qualitative methods are clearly in the ascendancy (Payne *et al.*, 2004).

Peace in our times?

Although the paradigm wars have cut deeply into the sociological landscape, there is growing dissatisfaction with the once orthodox view that quantitative and qualitative methods are rooted in incompatible ontological and epistemological commitments. Indeed it has become fairly commonplace for methods text books to drive home the point that distinctions between quantitative and qualitative methods are neither absolute nor clear-cut (Bryman, 2004; Silverman, 2001; Gilbert, 2008; see also Hammersley, 1992; Oakley, 1999). Some commentators have even pointed to a new 'methodological pluralism', based on tolerance of a variety of methods which extends either side of the 'dubious' dichotomy between quantitative and qualitative methods, though this pluralism is said to be both incomplete and rarely evident in mixed methods approaches (Payne *et al.*, 2004).

The arguments in favour of methodological pluralism are important from our perspective because they underpin the approach we have used to study suicide. Outlining the basic rationale for pluralism, Bryman (1988) argues that differences between quantitative and qualitative methods are largely technical, rather than epistemological, and that choices between them should be made on the basis of what is appropriate to the research question rather than prior commitments to a particular paradigm (see also Bell and Newby, 1977; Bell and Roberts, 1984). While maintaining that differences between these types of method are 'overblown', Bryman does not completely reject the distinction between them, nor does he entirely abandon the paradigms perspective. Rather, he retains the quantitative/qualitative distinction 'because it represents a useful means of classifying different methods of social research and because it is a helpful umbrella for a range of issues concerned with the practice of social research' (Bryman, 2004: 19). Quantitative and qualitative research are said to represent distinct research strategies, which differ over the role of theory as well as in terms of their epistemological and ontological commitments. But these distinctions are not 'hard-and-fast' and constitute tendencies rather than definitive connections. Both quantitative research and qualitative research can involve elements that are more typically associated with the other, so that quantitative research can contain elements of interpretivism and qualitative research can take an objectivist orientation and be geared towards hypothesis testing.

Once the quantitative/qualitative distinction ceases to be treated as a rigid one then the benefits of mixed strategy research become fairly obvious. Simply put, these different methods can be repositioned so that they become complimentary, rather than oppositional, with each being used to compensate for the limitations of the other. The net result is a fuller multi-dimensional representation that attends to both elements of the commonly drawn sociological dichotomies. There are various ways in which different methods may be combined within a multi-strategy approach. Among the best known are triangulation whereby quantitative research is used to corroborate qualitative findings or vice versa; facilitation where one research strategy is used to aid the other; and complementarity where both strategies are used to ensure that different aspects of an investigation can be dovetailed (Hammersley, 1996). Our approach is closest to complementarity and approximates to what Bryman calls 'filling in the gaps', which occurs 'when the researcher cannot rely on either a quantitative or qualitative method alone and must buttress his or her findings with a method drawn from the other research strategy' (2004: 458).

A dual paradigms approach

We are broadly sympathetic with Bryman's position and have sought to be consistent with the open, flexible approach he advocates. While seeking to transcend the frequently posited divide between quantitative and qualitative strategies we have found it useful to retain something like a paradigms perspective, albeit one that recognises the blurred edges involved. Qualitative methods were placed at the forefront of our approach as a corrective to the overwhelmingly quantitative orientation of suicidology and because we take seriously the interpretive critique developed by the likes of Douglas (1967) and Atkinson (1978), though we do not, ultimately, reach the same conclusions as them. Suicide is a peculiarly slippery construct and the interpretative aspects involved provide an important focus for our study. We wanted to both examine what we know about suicidal lives *and* take a critical stance on the knowledge itself. This required a necessarily broad view of the 'social context of suicide', which included the social construction of knowledge.

The detailed empirical analysis presented in the following chapters is based on coroners' case files of officially recorded suicides. What was found in the files has been treated as both a *topic* and a *resource* because insights were sought into two different dimensions of reality. The first dimension concerned the way evidence is constructed by all parties (both living and now dead) and the second concerned the substance of the evidence we have about the circumstances, beliefs and actions of suicidal individuals. This two pronged approach is, we believe, a sociological necessity because the social context of suicide involves processes of sense-making, which are evident in the way knowledge about suicide is constructed by professional and lay actors, as well as the material circumstances of the suicidal individual (insofar as they can be recovered). Juxtaposing objectivism and constructionism in this way provides part of the basis on which we lay claim to a dual para-digms approach and echoes something of Fine's (1997, 2007; after Gubrium [1993]) notion of 'cautious naturalism'. Working on the his-torical construction of social problems, Fine argues that for strict con-structionists to reject the possibility of studying objective structural conditions is a form of 'ontological hopelessness' (1997: 298) and for sociologists to 'ignore the effects of social structure is to deny their birthright' (1997: 317). A cautious naturalism, he explains, 'recognizes that confident knowledge and interpretive schemata both contribute to our learning from the past' (Fine, 2007: 33). Applying this principle to our study, we believe it is possible to use coroners' files to make some moderatum generalisations (Payne and Williams, 2005) about the social structural context of suicide. If, for example, the breakdown of a relationship is cited as significant in a suicide note as well as by friends and family of the deceased then we can reasonably conclude that it was an important part of the suicide's social context. If there are gendered features of the reaction to the relationship breakdown, as described in the inquest evidence, then we can reasonably make some connection to social structure. We must also accept that evidence about relationship breakdown is constructed on the basis of various common sense theories about relationships and about suicides, though we might also add that such assumptions are part of the repertoire of knowledge available to suicidal individuals (Canetto, 1992–93) and should, therefore, be taken seriously.

While making use of both quantitative and qualitative strategies, we have not sought to mix our methods in the sense of interweaving them. Each mode of analysis was conducted largely separately from the other and this is reflected in the way they have been presented. Our interpretation of the quantitative findings was sensitised by an appreciation of our qualitative analysis and additional qualitative work was carried out to further explore the main quantitative findings, but even here the two types of analysis have been presented separately (see Chapter 7). By maintaining such methodological distinctions our analysis retains something of a paradigms approach, with each approach being used according to its strengths. Qualitative analysis attends to the details of each case and is sensitive to both meaning and the processual nature of the circumstances surrounding suicide, though, in isolation, there is a danger that such an approach might lose sight of the structural dimensions involved. Quantitative analysis, by contrast, is better suited to identifying regularities and patterns within the dataset, providing a general outline of the material conditions that shape and structure suicidal behaviour. This mode of analysis is pivotal to our approach because it provides a framework for considering aetiological questions. The disadvantage of quantitative techniques is that they tend to reify 'variables' and provide a rather static one-dimensional perspective which is unable to penetrate the depth of the meanings involved (numeric data are, after all, abbreviated terms of reference for a fuzzy messy reality). The key point, then, is that we need both forms of analysis, with each being read in light of the other. By treating quantitative and qualitative readings as complimentary parts of a unified whole it is possible to transcend the core sociological dichotomies that are drawn between the individual and the social, the agential and the structural, and so on.

Our approach owes much to Bourdieu's thinking as outlined in the previous chapter, though we have sought to take account of some of the criticisms of his social praxeology. Bourdieu's use of statistics has been described as 'a little cavalier' and is said to reveal 'a residual positivism' (Jenkins, 1992: 60). As well as being overconfident that his statistics represented that which they purported to represent, Bourdieu has been criticised for failing to recognise that much of his survey data

were synoptic presentations of respondents' accounts of their prefer-
ences and habits etc. Our approach, by contrast, starts from a constructionist perspective and builds towards a more objectivist approach
which uses social actors' representations as the raw material through
which the workings of the external social world may be recovered.
This process of recovery, we argue, can be achieved by identifying
patterns and regularities in social actors' collective representations.
Once such patterns and regularities have been identified, social actors'
immediate lived experience should, as Bourdieu advocated, be reintroduced to explicate the categories of perception and appreciation that
structure their actions (see Chapter 7).

A sociological autopsy approach to suicide research

Psychological autopsy studies form an important and well-established
tradition within suicidology. Such studies focus on individual cases
and are conducted post-mortem, usually by psychiatrists or psychologists. Their aim is typically to measure risk factors among a relatively
small sample of cases. We refer to our approach as a 'sociological
autopsy' in conscious mimicry of the disciplinary claim of the psychological autopsy, but with a view to exploring the possibilities of socio-
logically-oriented research on individual suicides. Sociologists have
traditionally viewed the study of individual cases as irredeemably
psychological and, following Durkheim, have tended to concentrate
on suicide rates. Part of Durkheim's case against the study of individual suicides has arguably been proved wrong by evidence from
psychiatric and psychological studies which shows that a high proportion of suicides feature mental illness, often undiagnosed (see
Cavanagh, Carson, Sharpe and Lawrie, 2003). In contrast to the dominant tradition of research on suicide rates, we emphasise the sociological value of qualitatively-driven mixed method research (Mason,
2006) on *individual* cases for generating insights into the social context
in which they occur.

We are not the first to use the term 'sociological autopsy', though
it is not routinely applied to suicide research. The best known example
of a 'social autopsy' is that conducted by Klinenberg (2002) in his
study of deaths during the 1995 Chicago Heat Wave. Klinenberg's
approach has proved controversial in some quarters, prompting a heated
methodological debate in *American Sociological Review*. Klinenberg

sought to enhance existing knowledge from individual-level public health research on the 739 heat wave deaths by focusing on area effects and his analysis attracted considerable attention from both the media and academics in the US. The study employed a multiple research strategy, involving, amongst other things, fieldwork in specific neighbourhoods and observation in a newsroom. Data on individual deaths came primarily from Public Administrators' office files of unclaimed personal belongings from people who died alone, a database from the Medical Examiner's Office and police reports on the circumstances in which bodies were discovered, alongside several life histories. On the basis of these data, one of the book's chapters highlights the impact of social deprivation in a predominantly African-American neighbourhood, North Lawndale, with the isolation of elders being linked to a degraded physical environment and the fear of crime which caused people to stay indoors.

Duneier (2006) criticises Klinenberg for not enquiring sufficiently into the individual deaths in North and South Lawndale, accusing him of committing the ecological fallacy by extrapolating to individual circumstances from area-level data. Further enquiries by Duneier and his team led to the apparent discovery that most of the residents of North Lawndale who died in the heat wave had not been living alone, many of them were not 'elders' and many had drug or alcohol problems. Klinenberg (2006) has vigorously defended his conclusions, dismissing the neighbours' accounts that Duneier uses as unreliable, being based on decade-old retrospection and hearsay, and Klinenberg re-asserted his claims about people dying alone on the basis of ethnographic evidence. He has also challenged the significance of any drug or alcohol misuse to the deaths of these individuals on the basis of checking against the Medical Examiner's reports and has hit back at Duneier, accusing him of 'quick-hit' ethnography.

We summarise this debate in order to locate our approach. We have not attempted, as Klinenberg did, to locate deaths within the ecology of local areas, due partly to considerations of anonymity – choosing from the outset not to identify the location of the study – and because of resource limitations. The data in coroners' files on social class and ethnicity were also sparse, placing further limitations on our sociological reflections. We did not check the witness statements that were in the files by interviewing significant others as Duneier recommends. To do so with a large enough sample for statistical analysis would be a considerable challenge, though we agree it is desirable. All this is to acknowledge what could be seen as the limitations of our approach, though there are also things to be said in its defence. In many ways, our approach falls somewhere between Klinenberg's macro-level analysis and the ethnographic approach recommended by Duneier. We have drawn on individual-level data which include, in most cases, the testimonies of several witnesses who knew the deceased well. We also have data for every case on the circumstances in which the body was found. Ours is a reasonably large and robust data set compared to most qualitative research, moreover, and we can claim to be extending the methodological options for social autopsy through our efforts to develop a dual paradigms approach. We seek to show that social autopsy data can be used to study the social construction of death, whilst also providing the basis for reasonably objective conclusions about the social circumstances of individuals in life and death.

References to 'sociological autopsy' can be found in the work of Chatterjee and Bailey (1993) and Slater (2005), though only the latter uses the term in relation to suicide. Owens *et al.* (2008) also apply qualitative approaches to study suicide and generate important sociological insights, but they retain the term 'psychological autopsy'. While mainstream psychological autopsy studies do seem to leave room for a social focus, Cavanagh *et al.*'s (2003) systematic review found that such studies contain limited evidence on psycho-social factors. Our analysis can help to fill this gap by taking a consciously sociological approach. In contrast to mainstream psychological autopsy studies, we believe it is important to recognise the inevitably interpretive dimension involved and this has led us to a qualitatively-driven approach, which allows for case-based as well as variable-based analysis. Our approach also reflects a desire to retain the multi-dimensional complexity of individual cases and a reluctance to reduce any sociological analysis to a mono-causal interpretation. There is a parallel here with what Sibeon (1999) calls 'anti-reductionist sociology'. His is not a post-modernist approach with a focus on fragmentation, but aims to consolidate a complex mix of social explanations. This is an aim we share, though we recognise that our attempts to encompass tensions and even contradictions in data, rather than eliminate them, may have resulted in a messy, rather than smooth, account (Law, 2004).

The data

Our analysis is based on officially recorded cases of suicide. A team of three researchers read a sample of 100 suicide case files selected from a single coroner's office in the UK covering a medium-sized city, an adjacent rural area and an industrial town. The sample was made up of the first 100 suicide verdicts we encountered from 2002 onwards and stretched over a three-year period. For reasons of anonymity we are not naming the geographical area, but we can note that, in terms of age and sex profiles, the selected cases are broadly similar to recorded suicides in England and Wales as a whole: the ratio of male suicides to female was just under 4:1 and the average age was 46 years (44 for males, 53 for females). The city which makes up the biggest part of the population of the study district has a minority ethnic population a little above the UK average of 7.9 per cent, but there were insufficient data on ethnicity in the coroners' files to allow for its inclusion in the data analysis. Indicators of social class, such as occupation, were also partial or missing in many cases. The data contained in the case files came from a diverse range of sources and to consider documentary research as mono-method in this context would be inaccurate. Files included forms filled out by the coroner; scribbles by the coroner on file wallets; police statements from witnesses and significant others; forensic pathology reports; medical letters and reports, especially psychiatric ones; suicide notes; mobile phone records; photographs of corpses; letters to the coroner and newspaper clippings. These data are so diverse in terms of the conditions under which they were designed and produced that, taken together, they can arguably be seen as a 'multi-modal' data set (Fincham *et al.*, 2007). The main sources of data were as follows:

i.   *Suicide notes* are generally written in conditions of extreme anxiety and distress in the period immediately before death. This writing is preserved in the original and from the coroner's perspective must not be tampered with. The production of the notes varies considerably, with messages being left in envelopes on the dashboard of the car containing a suicide victim, taped to the door of a bathroom in a hotel where somebody had killed themselves, left on tables in the same room as the body, in rooms away from the body or slipped under friends' doors. There were messages left on personal computers, retrieved mobile telephone text messages and scrawled notes left on beds. The notes are also written with particular audiences in mind and anticipate some of the reactions that might be expected to the suicide. There are some common aspects of design, including (often, but not always) apologies to specific individuals, explanation of reasons for the suicide and instructions for a funeral or disposal of possessions. Chapter 5 is dedicated to a discussion of the social meaning of suicide notes.

ii.   *Interviews with relatives and friends of the deceased* take the form of written witness statements and originate as spoken accounts, but are subject to remediation by police officers and codified in professional language to meet the needs of the court. Statements are usually taken shortly after the discovery of a suicide and are a mix of factual and emotive statements. They often contain details about the recent past, the state of mind of the deceased and key events in his or her life that may have contributed to the eventual suicide. The orientation of these statements towards the perceived needs of the legal process (mediated by police officers) results in a formula (or 'grammar') that should perhaps be seen as a 'mode of regulation' (Kress and Van Leeuwen, 2001: 22). There are some familiar elements of narrative that tend to reappear quite often, including reflection on the deceased's trajectory of happiness/depression, the events leading up to the death, the last exchange the witness had with the deceased and so on. These statements do contain corporeal detail, as it is often these people that first encounter the bodies. However, it appears in our sample that the majority of people that find bodies remove themselves from the scene and seek help from someone else, a neighbour or the emergency services. It is the witness statements from the friends and relatives that are used to provide an historical context to the death to assist the coroner in reaching a verdict. The level of detail contained in these statements varies widely, from very sparse comment to pages of detailed accounts of the life of the deceased.

iii.   *Interviews with eye witnesses* are also subject to remediation by police officers and describe the circumstances surrounding the death and its aftermath. Bodies are discovered by close family members, by people who knew the deceased but were not members of the family and also by people who did not know the deceased, but who just happened to be around when the suicide occurred. Eye witnesses who are unknown to the deceased have fallen into at least three categories (see below). Again, since these statements are conveyed via conventions of police recording, they are structured by a clear 'grammar of design', to use Kress and Van Leeuwen's (2001) terminology.

(1) Members of the general public

These witnesses have simply happened upon the suicide. They include hotel chambermaids coming across bodies in rooms, people walking their dogs and coming across a body hanging and passers-by witnessing someone jumping in a river. Just occasionally an expression of powerful emotion ends up in a witness statement, but because of their primary legal role as evidence of the means of death, these statements rarely convey any shock or horror. One would imagine that in many cases, as with close friends and relatives, a fairly emotional account becomes recorded by police officers as a rather detached description of body location and condition, because of evidential priorities.

(2) Police Officers

The police are often called when someone – a family member, neighbour, or passer-by – notices that something is amiss, for example a suicide note has been discovered by a relative and the house is locked and the police are called to break in. These statements are very explicitly couched in the institutional language of police procedure.

(3) Paramedics

Paramedic statements involve additional formulas for describing medical procedures carried out on the deceased. Occasionally they convey a tone of professional defensiveness – perhaps anticipating complaint or litigation where the suicidal individual might conceivably have been kept alive through paramedic intervention.

iv. *Pathology reports* are inevitably clinical in their content, containing details of the size, weight and condition of major organs and any physical trauma suffered. These accounts can be distressing to read in a very different way from the more personal accounts of friends and relatives. The level of detail about often horrific injuries is reported in such a way as to accentuate the dissection of the body. Again these reports reveal a clear grammar of design, with the same headings and sub-headings appearing in almost every report and considerable repetition between reports of the same anatomical and pharmacological terminology.

v. *Psychiatric and psychological reports* often chart the emotional collapse of the deceased and occasionally reveal elements of personalities or relationships not mentioned by, and perhaps not known to, relatives or friends. It should be pointed out that there are differences in the statements between psychiatrists, who will often catalogue reactions to drug prescription regimes, and psychologists who tend to focus more on reactions to life events or significant relationships. As with the other professional reports noted above, there are occupational grammars of design, although psychiatric and psychological reports are less formulaic than those of pathologists. As with paramedic reports, there are occasionally reports that are constructed in anticipation of possible complaints. These contain considerable detail of the chronology of appointments and treatments offered.

Ethical considerations

Suicide is a highly sensitive topic and any suicide research which is not based on data which are already anonymised requires careful consideration in terms of what constitutes ethical conduct. There are particular challenges of anonymity for qualitative research on suicide cases, given the detailed accounts this research can involve. For this study we had permission from the coroner to read suicide case files. We did not seek permission from family members of the deceased. We took this decision on the basis that the file concerned an individual who was now deceased and therefore not available to consent to the study. It is not possible to ascertain without this individual's view which family member would be the most appropriate person from whom to seek permission. There were difficult family relationships in some of these cases and it was therefore potentially problematic to approach family members who the deceased themselves might not have regarded as having the right to give or withhold access to the file. We decided to read the files on the basis of the coroner's permission but to maintain anonymity by not recording any identifiable information about the deceased; not identifying the location of the coroner's office other than to say it was in 'the UK'; and generalising or disguising biographical details, such as making minor changes to age and occupation. Any such changes were in keeping with the social location of the individual. We accept that it was not an ethically straightforward decision to proceed on the basis of the coroner's permission alone and another research team may have taken a different view, however we were satisfied on balance with the ethical basis of the decision we took.

Decisions about ethical research have practical consequences. So the decision to mask the location of the coroner's office meant it was not possible to consider the social characteristics of the areas in which the deceased had lived, as was the case, for example, in Klinenberg's (2002) research on the Chicago heat wave. Another ethical issue was care of the researchers. Reading the files could be upsetting and we tried to ensure that there was a de-briefing opportunity for the researchers after time spent with the case files (see Fincham *et al.*, 2008). The research was approved by a multi-centre National Health Service research ethics committee.

Making sense of Coroners' files

There are, of course, potential difficulties in relying on coroners' records. There can be variations between coroners as to which cases are given a verdict of 'suicide' and which are given 'open' verdicts. Based on ethnographic research with medical examiners, the nearest equivalent to coroners in the USA, Timmermans (2005) argued that under-reporting of suicides can be explained by the very professional characteristics that protect the medical examiners' authority, namely the insistence on legal thresholds, the privileging of pathological evidence and maintenance of close relationships with law enforcement and medical personnel. As part of our field work, we visited two neighbouring coroners' offices, to interview the coroner and read ten files from each place. This satisfied us that the kinds of evidence used were broadly similar to those in our main research site. While we did not seek to address differences of interpretation between coroners, recent research does indicate that official records retain a certain validity (see Chapter 1) and that using data from a single coroner is justifiable. Based on their study of practice in England and Wales during the 1950s to 1970s, for example, Sainsbury and Jenkins (1982) argued that errors in reporting deaths were randomised and therefore made no difference to comparisons within and between countries. While Pescosolido and Mendelsohn (1986) found systematic misreporting of suicide in the USA, they concluded that this had little impact on the variables commonly used to test sociological theories of suicide.

Our reading of the research led us to an epistemologically pragmatic position. We accept that evidence about suicide, including documents in coroners' files, is produced under specific conditions which affect how it should be read, but maintain that such evidence aims to establish something about an externally verifiable social world. Although it may only ever approximate to what actually happened, we believe that evidence presented to a Coroner, including suicide notes and statements by relatives of the victim and witnesses, provides a reasonable basis for making tentative judgements about the social circumstances of a suicide. That said, we acknowledge our approach is limited in some important respects. We have, as already noted, relied on a single Coroner's office and the possibility of idiosyncrasies remains. Our sample of 100 cases is, moreover, a small one for the purposes of statistical generalisation, though psychological autopsy studies typically have even smaller samples. A study of this kind, then, is neither a very in-depth study of a handful of cases nor a population-level epidemiological analysis. Our conclusions are, therefore, necessarily tentative and open to refutation or confirmation by future research.

Data were generated from coroners' files using what was an essentially qualitative approach. Case files were read by the fieldwork team, a coding scheme was agreed and cases (rather than excerpts) were thematically coded using N-vivo version 2.0. As is often the case with qualitative research, the coding and classification system was developed through contact with the data rather than being designed to test prior hypotheses. Initial codes indicated whether or not the contents of a case file made reference to a particular social or behavioural factor. Any indication from the file of, for example, bereavement, debt or drug/alcohol problems was coded accordingly. Although the analysis was inductive, the amount of data in the files meant decisions had to be made about what to record and our attention was inevitably drawn to factors which frequently reoccurred and/or are well-known from the epidemiological literature on suicide. The data collection included a combination of the researchers' own notes and verbatim data excerpts, some of which were quite lengthy. In a sense, then, the process of analysis was begun while the data were being collected.

Where initial coding revealed interesting themes for further exploration, we returned to the data to consider key themes in more depth. This process can be illustrated with reference to a specific example. One theme that was strongly evident from the files, and is also well-known from epidemiological research, concerned the role of relationship breakdown and this prompted further consideration on our part.

While the initial coding scheme simply indicated whether there was any mention of relationship breakdown, we returned to the case files in an attempt to develop a better appreciation of its impact. Where relationship breakdown was mentioned we sought to assess its relative importance to the suicidal act, as far as it was possible to gauge from the files. This involved identifying those cases where relationship breakdown seemed to be the main trigger, by which we mean it seemed to precipitate the suicidal act. Such acts usually occur in the context of several compounding social and psychological problems, and those cases where relationship breakdown was the main trigger did not necessarily depart from this general trend, but seemed to involve a clear connection between relationship breakdown and the decision to die. For these cases we also sought to categorise the apparent response of the suicidal individual to the relationship difficulties in terms of the social meanings of suicidal actions, with categories including punishment, over-dependence and separation from children (see Chapter 7).

The analysis was primarily based on conventional qualitative techniques with some supporting use of quantitative methods. Once a coding frame had been agreed and cases had been thematically coded using N-vivo software, the tabular coding profile was exported into SPSS for statistical analysis. Quantifying qualitative data in this way may be objectionable to some, but we were careful to agree a coding frame (based on initial analysis) which was systematically applied to the 100 cases, with cross-checking between coders. The main advantage of the quantitative analysis was that it enabled us to identify patterns and relationships between variables in a way that would have been difficult with a purely qualitative approach. Added to this, the analysis was conducted in a way that blurred the boundaries between quantitative and qualitative approaches. Although statistical techniques were used, they were applied in a way that was consistent with what are often held to be the defining characteristics of a qualitative approach: the analysis was highly exploratory and largely inductive in the sense that the emphasis was firmly on generating, rather than testing, hypotheses.

Suicide and the double hermeneutic

'Sociology', notes Giddens, 'is not concerned with a "pre-given" universe of objects, but with one which is constituted or produced by the active doings of subjects' (1976: 160). In this regard it differs markedly from the natural sciences which deal with a universe that is constituted 'as an object world independently of human existence' (1976: 160). One of the defining characteristics of sociology, then, is that it deals with a universe that has already been rendered meaningful by social actors themselves, and then reinterprets these meanings in terms of its own theoretical schemes. As such, sociological concepts are said to obey what Giddens (1976) describes as a 'double hermeneutic'. Our attempt to make sense of suicide clearly conforms to this principle because the case files included various explanations from the social actors involved, including the suicidal individual, witnesses, friends and relatives, professionals on the scene and, ultimately, the coroner. Rarely, if ever, could the 'facts' of the case simply be read off the file and this raises important questions about the relationship between 'common sense' understanding and sociological accounts. To illustrate the possibilities and limitations of the sociological autopsy approach we will show how suicide records are shaped by 'common sense' theorising and the interests of the living. We will also consider two cases in detail to demonstrate the complexity of the circumstances surrounding suicide. Our intention here is not to develop any major empirical claims, but simply to outline the potential of the sociological autopsy approach and to consider how we might best manage the hermeneutic requirement.

The files were replete with 'common sense' theories about suicide, which contained several points of contact with academic explanations. There is, for example, a well-established association between financial problems and men's suicides (Canetto, 1997; Kushner, 1993), which was reflected in the files. To illustrate its currency as a common sense explanation, we saw a case where financial problems were cited as relevant to a male suicide by one of the witnesses, even though there was no other evidence to support a connection and the reported views of the deceased made no reference to money matters. In case 18, the father of the deceased (male, age 26) begins his statement thus: 'Jack[1] up to a week before the incident had had financial worries regarding a car he had purchased approximately 8 months earlier.' Other evidence indicated that this suicide was

---

[1]All names are pseudonyms.

prompted by Jack having been due to meet his ex-girlfriend for a drink and her not turning up. We do not mean to suggest that the father was wrong to cite financial worries as being relevant to the case and we readily acknowledge the complexity of the social circumstances surrounding most suicides. The weight of the evidence suggests that financial worries were not the only, or even the main, trigger, however, and may have been cited because of a common sense assumption that this is an understandable reason for a suicide, especially for males, perhaps, given the continuing cultural association between men and work/money.

Relationship breakdown was also cited as a common sense justification for suicide in the eyes of inquest witnesses, especially, it seems, for men, and this explanation is, again, consistent with the research evidence (see Stack, 2000b). We can see from the files *in situ* theorising by police officers whose accounts often mention failed relationships, whether or not this proves to be relevant in the evidence provided by other witnesses. Also, when visiting another local coroner's office (not our main site) we were told by the coroner's secretary that the suicides in her district were 'mostly young boys who've split up with their girlfriends'. In fact the picture for England and Wales shows that suicide rates are higher in mid-life and old age than in youth (see Chapter 7) and this district did not depart from the general trend. The secretary's summary of suicide trends reveals a popular preoccupation with the problem of suicides in young men, as shown in media reporting, but there is perhaps a newer focus in the popular imagination on men's responses to relationship breakdowns. Certainly, it is an association that fits with portrayals of suicide in popular culture, with failed relationships predominating in films featuring suicides for example (Agerbo *et al.*, 2009).

Relationship breakdown coupled with conflicts over children seems to be taken to be an especially understandable reason for suicides in men – understandable perhaps in the context of popular perceptions that family courts 'favour' women as carers of children and the angry politics of fatherhood, with fathers' rights groups citing suicides among separated fathers as evidence of the supposed cruelty of the judicial system. Case 30 (male, aged 32) was a very thin file with little evidence at all. Pretty much all we found out about the man is that he had been involved in a custody battle over his children aged five, eight and ten and was concerned about his ex-partner's care of them. We were told he had been due in court when he killed himself. This seemed to be a case where the coroner and his staff assumed it should be a straightforward 'suicide' verdict because of the custody battle – straightforward enough that little evidence was needed. The single explanation was stated in fairly stark terms in the evidence from witnesses, including those who knew him well, suggesting that the apparent cause 'made sense' to those lay and professional people who were assessing the death.

As well as acknowledging that evidence in case files is based on taken-for-granted assumptions about reasonable cause, we have to consider that the concerns of the living feature in the case files as much as those of the dead (see Chapter 4). This dynamic draws attention to the complexity of evidence about individual cases and the inevitably interpretive dimension of suicide research. As with psychological autopsy studies, decisions have to be taken by researchers in the field because the data cannot simply be assumed to speak for themselves. Although the files contained plenty of evidence of relationship breakdown being a significant factor in suicides, for example, they also contained some significant silences in this regard. In some cases partners deny any tensions, but other witnesses, such as friends of the deceased, clearly state that relationship difficulties were cited by the deceased as being amongst the principal triggers for the suicide. Case 41 was a self-employed man in the property business and there was some indication in the file of work-related stress. The police seemed to focus on debt as a possible understandable reason for suicide, while the man's secretary told the police her boss was reasonably happy, although he did experience stress and had a drink problem. The best clue to what may have been an important trigger was provided by a friend, who would not give a formal statement, but said that the girlfriend of the deceased was having an affair and that the victim had only learned this information on the night he died. The girlfriend herself made no mention of any affair. In Case 48, several witnesses reported that the context of the suicide was divorce, following domestic violence. The ex-wife provided detailed evidence, including the no doubt difficult admission that on the day before her former husband died, when he drunkenly talked of killing himself, she and her daughter had left him on his own 'as he had used this type of behaviour in the past to seek attention from family members'. What she did not mention was any difficulty her ex had with her new partner, even though he took an overdose on the day she had arranged for them all to socialise together.

What then are we to make of the common sense explanations and silences contained in the coroner's case files? According to Giddens (1976), sociologists cannot make social life available as a phenomenon for observation without drawing upon their everyday knowledge of it and, in this respect, they are no different from any other member of society. 'Mutual knowledge', Giddens explains, represents the interpretive schemes which both sociologists and laymen must use to make sense of social activity. This is reminiscent of the postulate of adequacy forwarded by Schutz (1953), which requires that social scientific concepts be constructed in a way that is understandable to the social actors involved. But Giddens maintains that the link between everyday knowledge and sociological knowledge does not simply flow in one direction as Schutz seems to suggest. Rather, 'there is continual "slippage" of the concepts constructed in sociology, whereby they are appropriated by those whose conduct they were originally coined to analyse, and hence tend to become integral features of that conduct' (Giddens, 1976: 162). Given the links between everyday knowledge and sociological knowledge, our general position is that the interpretations of social actors who are close to the deceased should not be dismissed as 'only' common sense, but should be treated as the building blocks from which sociological theory can be constructed. The stock of knowledge that inquest witnesses draw on about distress and what might reasonably make someone feel suicidal, it seems to us, is broadly the same as that which suicidal individuals draw on when experiencing distress.

Silences are, perhaps, more challenging, though they highlight the need for an interpretive dimension. Suicide is, perhaps, uniquely able to induce feelings of guilt in others and giving evidence to an inquest is, in some senses, a moral project. That witnesses may control the flow of information when giving such evidence is hardly surprising given the moral judgements that follow suicides and the connection between morality and responsibility (see, for example, Coyle and MacWhannell, 2002). Those who were close to someone who has died by suicide have to negotiate the hovering responsibility (Owens *et al.*, 2008), perhaps by minimising their own connection to any distress experienced by the deceased, or at least drawing certain lines around their own role. Interpreting inquest evidence, therefore, requires a critical stance on the available sources and a consideration of witnesses' positionality and expectations of audience.

Limitations and possibilities

We consider two examples of case-based analysis at this point to demonstrate the limitations and possibilities of our sociological autopsy approach. Firstly, we describe the evidence about Jane's life and death (Case 42) to illustrate the complexity of evidence and understanding that looking at individual suicide cases necessarily involves. Jane – not her real name – was a white woman, aged 32, who died in hospital having taken an overdose. She had left a suicide note in a prominent place for her house-mates to find, raising the possibility that she wanted to be stopped although it was also reported that she resisted the paramedics who tried to take her to hospital. The case file included statements from a male paramedic, male tenant 1, male tenant 2 and Jane's mother. There was also a post-mortem report from a forensic pathologist, a letter from the police to the coroner and a copy of the suicide note.

Table 3.1   Para-phrased Summary of Evidence about Jane (Case 42)

Paramedic: She was un-co-operative and refused treatment.

Tenant 1: She was a compulsive liar, paranoid, had a complex about her size, I think she invented a boyfriend and a miscarriage. When tenant 2 and I first moved in she tried to engage us in sexual encounters.

Tenant 2: (Similar to tenant 2 plus the following information) she got drunk on wine every night. She said she had a Bridget Jones lifestyle.

Mother: We had a perfect mother-daughter relationship. We would talk about everything. She helped care for her father before he died. We were in regular contact.

Post-mortem report: She died a day after admittance. There was no evidence of pregnancy.

Letter from police: She was depressed, low self-worth and relied on tenants for friendship.

Suicide note: I've got no-one. I'm a joke to you. You say everything is my fault. I do all the cooking and cleaning. Please look after the dogs. They and you will be better off without me. I've nothing to live for. I'm embarrassing. I'm unattractive. You criticise me all the time. My confidence has been shattered. People laugh at me because of the way I look. I can't live with the guilt of losing the babies even though it wasn't anything I'd done. Don't tell my family about it.

The first thing to note is that these documents should be socially situated. Given the moral tone of suicide discourse noted above, the tenants will likely be trying to distance themselves from any responsibility for what has occurred. The paramedic might perhaps prioritise efficiently processing a patient and may be reflecting familiar organisational discourse about difficult individuals. All the statements have been processed by the police according to a fairly formulaic pattern, including only what they perceive necessary for legal purposes. This particular file is relatively detailed, though we have nothing from Jane before her last hours and we have little detail from her mother. There is, moreover, no-one else who can shed any light on whether or not Jane lied to her lodgers about having had a boyfriend and a miscarriage, although the pathologist's report would suggest that she had not been pregnant.

Is it possible to incorporate these very different accounts into an interpretation which does justice to them all? Jane's suicide note confirms a fairly stark picture of highly gendered pressure to do with body image, narrowly defined femininity and sexuality. She describes disrespectful treatment from the men she lived with. But to suggest that this is a case that can simply be understood in terms of the sociology of gender would be to miss an important psychological dimension. The note in the post-mortem report that there had been no sign of pregnancy suggests Jane may not have told the truth about having recently miscarried twins. There was a psychological frailty perhaps, albeit one that needs to be understood in the context of a sociological account of gender relations, but perhaps a frailty without which she may not have taken the overdose. The impact of gendered norms on this particular individual has to be understood, as far as is possible with very limited data, alongside her willingness to present as real something that seems to be objectively untrue. A psychiatric study might see indications of a personality disorder here and perhaps the best we can do is refer the case to a psychologist. Certainly, Jane's death does not sit neatly into the structurally located classification of suicide we present later (see Chapter 7), though the claims she makes about a boyfriend and miscarriage fit the general theme of loneliness, relationship breakdown and loss, albeit possibly imagined.

Our second example represents an attempt to move beyond an acknowledgement of complexity and 'mess' to illustrate the possibilities of the sociological autopsy approach. The aim here is to demonstrate coherence by highlighting what we regard to be the most salient aspects of the social context of the case in the light of the available evidence and the wider field of suicide and gender research. Mark (Case 7) was a 30-year-old man who killed himself by carbon monoxide poisoning in his car soon after a very serious suicide attempt by the same means. The social context of his case seems to include a toxic combination of spite to his ex-partner (the mother of his child) and anxiety about his public image.

A psychiatric report noted that Mark 'felt very humiliated, embarrassed and quite upset' about his previous suicide attempt. He had no prior history of psychiatric involvement and his embarrassment may well reflect gendered cultural scripts of suicidal behaviour. 'Successful' suicide tends to be masculinised, as decisive and requiring courage, whilst a 'failed' suicide attempt is often feminised, as weak and ambivalent (Canetto, 1995). Mark's reaction of embarrassment and humiliation can easily be understood in these terms as shame related to behaviour which is feminised. The file gave an impression of someone who was generally concerned about how he was seen by others. He had been imprisoned some years before his death for theft from an employer and told his best friend shortly before his death that he felt he had hurt his family. He further said that 'he felt he had built up an image to everyone that he could no longer live up to' (his best friend's statement as drafted by a police officer).

This explicit reference to 'image' is unusual, although similar issues may well be implicit in many male suicides. The idea of a man's 'image', viewed from the perspective of critical men's studies, connects with Connell's (1995) concept of 'hegemonic masculinity'. Although this concept has been criticised as suggesting 'the notion of a fixed (male) structure' (Whitehead, 2002: 94), Connell insists it refers to 'the circulation of models of admired masculine conduct' that do not 'correspond closely to the lives of the majority of men' but express 'ideals, fantasies and desires' (2002: 90). Similarly, Bourdieu emphasises the important role of honour in masculine domination, describing it as 'a system of demands which remains, in many cases, inaccessible' (2001: 50). Honour, shame and manliness all require public affirmation; they must be 'validated before other men' (2001: 52). Applying these ideas to a sociological understanding of gendered suicide, Scourfield (2005) has highlighted the tension that can be produced when a gap between aspiration and reality in suicidal men becomes absolutely overt and recognised, rather than submerged or socially embedded, and a life marked by a loss of masculine honour is not seen as worth living. As Mark wrote in one of his several suicide notes 'I Just wished that I was normal and Respectable instead of who I am'.

The public account Mark gave for his suicidal feelings rests on his failure to conform to a respectable image and the debts he had accrued. Debt is perhaps an expected and even acceptable reason for suicidality in men, given the traditional association between masculinity and work, as noted earlier. Mark did hint to his best friend that there were 'more things in the pipeline that would become evident' (best friend's statement to police) and the suicide notes he left revealed a conflicted sense of anger directed towards his ex-partner. Mark wrote several notes, one of which was to his ex-partner who was the mother of his child although he specified that he did not want his family to know about this note in case it further upset them. He started the note to his ex-partner by writing 'if you are reading this letter I am no longer here thank God, no more thoughts of what a Spiteful bitch you are' and proceeded to write a note that was designed to cause her intense distress. He wrote 'make no mistakes this is because of you and nothing else' and went on to explain how difficult it should be for her to live with herself knowing she was responsible for his death. He carefully listed everyday events and objects that ought to remind her of him and cause her pain. He twice mentioned the potential impact on their son, again emphasising that she was responsible for this. In stark contrast, he left a note for the police and any person who found his body, apologising for any 'hassle' and leaving his name, address and details of next of kin.

In light of Mark's apparent preoccupation with how others saw him and a sense of respectability, we might speculate that the motive of punishing his ex-partner was apparently not mentioned to the best friend (or at least not mentioned in the friend's witness statement) because he was aware of possible moral censure, especially in relation to the impact on his young son. It was possible for Mark to be concerned about avoiding negative public reaction, to the extent of apologising to a stranger who might find his body, and simultaneously to carefully construct a suicide note to cause maximum anguish to his ex-partner. We do not have any data on the history of his relationship with any ex-partners, but we can arguably see in this case a similar dynamic that can be identified in some instances of domestic abuse of a concern with public respectability alongside simultaneous extremes of private abuse. Such extreme denigration of the ex-partner does suggest a personalised misogyny; not necessarily a generalised hatred of women, but a hatred of an ex-partner which is somehow allowable. While Mark did not want to make the hatred public, committing his thoughts to paper does, perhaps, suggest there is a social or cultural space allowed for such extreme views on an ex-partner.

Mark's case, like Jane's, makes reference to thwarted domestic ambitions, be they real or imagined, but while Jane's suicide is shrouded in possible personality disorder, Mark's seems to be much more immediately bound up with the structurally mediated currents of anomic failure and egoistic loss. In contrast to Jane's case, Mark's fits squarely into our structurally located classification of suicide (see Chapter 7). While interpretive dimensions are fundamental, human behaviour cannot be fully explained in terms of intentional action. What people do must also be understood as a set of 'occurrences', with structural properties (Giddens, 1976). As such, the strength of the approach we are recommending is that interpretive and structural readings compliment and clarify one another.

Conclusion

The epistemological and theoretical debates that Jamison noted in the quotation cited at the beginning of this chapter are still very much in evidence. In the course of the chapter we have introduced an approach to researching suicide which we believe draws on both the traditions within sociology that are more obviously allied to science and those that have more obvious affinities with the humanities. We have stated the case for a qualitatively-driven dual paradigms sociological autopsy approach, which mimics the psychological autopsy, but has an avowedly sociological purpose, both encompassing the construction of knowledge about suicide cases and also aiming towards reasonably objective judgements about the circumstances of suicidal individuals. Although the chapter is primarily methodological in focus, and does not seek to make any major empirical claims, we have briefly illustrated the application of the sociological autopsy approach, with particular reference to two cases that highlight the associated possibilities and limitations.

At several points in the chapter we have highlighted the complexity and messiness of the social circumstances that typically surround suicide, arguing we should seek to avoid reductionist mono-causal explanations. There is, we feel, a middle path to be negotiated between recognising complexity and seeking precision, which a dual paradigms approach potentially provides. Law's (2004) call for social science to preserve the messiness of data rather than creating artificially smooth accounts of social life is particularly pertinent to the study of suicide. There is, for example, more than one story to tell about Jane (Case 42, see above), and boiling down the evidence about her life and death to a simple clean conclusion does little to promote real understanding. That said, there remains, in our view, a strong epistemological and moral case for a generalising social science of suicide. Given the clear harms involved, there is a clear moral/ political imperative behind suicide prevention though such activities raise important ethical considerations. Circumventing another complex debate, we believe academic research has a responsibility to contribute to an ethically and socially desirable goal such as suicide prevention and this is where preserving messiness could be seen to have limitations. Embracing the possibility of different stories, as Law suggests, may help professionals working with suicidal individuals to understand the unavoidable uncertainty involved in such work – a possibility that we return to in Chapter 8. But this is only part of what is required. Recognising complexity does not have to mean retreating into a relativistic, anything goes, sociology-as-story telling. There is, as Kirk and Miller note, 'a world of empirical reality out there' and it 'does not tolerate all understandings' equally (1986: 11). Accessing this world is, of course, no easy matter and the best starting point, perhaps, is provided by a recognition of the inherent difficulties involved. After all, 'Science does not aspire to godlike certainty: that would be more characteristic of religious fanaticism. All it provides is the best explanations in the light of the available evidence' (Smith, 1994: 1046). It is to evidence that we now turn, in the first of a pair of broadly constructionist chapters which focus on the nature of the evidence in coroners' case files.

4
Suicide Case Files as Sites of Identity Creation

In this chapter we want to use the artefacts that constitute the inquest file to draw out some of the assumptions inherent in the inquest process regarding documents and identities. Specifically, we are concerned with relationships: how they extend into documents and how they constitute different kinds of persons and identities, during someone's lifetime and beyond. We will do so by drawing on recent ethnographic approaches to the study of documents (Riles, 2006a) and of the lifecycle (Hallam *et al.*, 1999; Hockey and Draper, 2005). This emphasis on continued connections may at first appear surprising as death tends to be conceptualised as a severing of relationships and an end to existence. Indeed, the inquest process itself is framed as a precondition to achieving closure by establishing the medical causes of death and the circumstances leading up to it. For instance, until the inquest has been completed, no final certificate of death can be issued. Yet we suggest that this official inquiry into the causes and circumstances of a sudden death also creates a space in which social identities are scrutinised, redefined and challenged, and involves the acquisition of new identities beyond the life-course (Hockey and Draper, 2005).

A conception of personhood as beginning before birth and extending after death presupposes a relational approach, wherein personhood is not possessed, but is generated and performed through interactions with other agents, human and non-human, alive and dead (Strathern, 1992). It is a focus on persons as created through a multiplicity of relationships that allows us to study inquest documents not only as objects *per se*, but as extension of and co-creators in the generation of different kinds of social identities. In relation to the deceased in the context of suicide inquests, such a distributive understanding of personhood raises a number of issues. First, identities and agency have long been recognised as embodied, but how are they affected by death? Second, if the identities of the living are multiple and often contradictory, what happens to these identities when a person dies? Finally, if identities are situated in relations, what are the implications for the connections between the living and the dead? When addressing these questions we will pay particular attention to the evidence from various actors that is presented to coroners in suicide cases rather than on the judgements of coroners themselves. After introducing our theoretical framework, we will sketch the conditions in which we encountered the suicide records and proceed by focusing on the following artefacts collated in the files: reports by medical scientists, health professionals, and physicians as well as witness statements by relatives, friends, and members of the public. We will only briefly touch on suicide notes here, as they will be discussed in detail in the following chapter.

Drawing on ethnographic approaches to files and to the life-course

Hockey and Draper (2005) have argued for a reconfiguration of our understanding of the theoretical concept of the life-course. They maintain that, particularly through artefacts, identities extending before birth and beyond death are created, or in their words: 'Around bones, photos and bootees, personal and military histories are built; and family lives are dreamed into being' (Hockey and Draper, 2005: 54).

Hallam *et al.* (1999) suggest, in similar fashion and as a challenge to mainstream sociological theorising about the body, that the construction of social identities does not in fact require the presence of a living body. On the basis of our research on suicide, we agree with these arguments, up to a point. Suicide inquest files, we propose, should be added to Hockey and Draper's list of artefacts through which social identities are able to continue well after death.

Moreover, on the basis of our research, we want to make four comments that are pertinent to the arguments of Hallam *et al.* and Hockey and Draper. First, through their death, the deceased can also acquire new identities, such as the official label of someone who has killed him or herself or the private one of someone who was unable to cope. Secondly, the identities of the deceased are not any less tangled up or confusing than those of the living. In the suicide files, different identities of the deceased jostled with each other, for instance as patients, parents, spouses, and as individual men or women, as they present themselves and are represented through patient files, witness statements and suicide notes. Thirdly, because of the distributed nature of personhood, the identities assigned to the deceased simultaneously give account of the concerns of the living. This also entails that the movement of identities is not one-way, but rather that the living are implicated in the identities of the dead. Finally, in the absence of the body as agent, the question of the authenticity of the identities of the deceased gains new significance. We propose that it is this constellation of absent bodies and multiple and contested identities, that opens the space for the debates surrounding a death by suicide to continue long after the inquest has closed.

The other body of work we are engaging with here concerns the ethnographic approach to the study of documents as developed by Annelise Riles. Her interests in documents first developed while working with Fijian bureaucrats and activists preparing for and participating in the United Nations Fourth World Conference on Women (Riles, 2001). Realising that her 'subject' – the elucidation, appreciation, presentation, and use of information – was as much part of the knowledge practices of her field site as it was of the social science tradition she was part of, Riles asked what this symmetry meant for ethnographic research whose claims to expertise were traditionally premised on an ability to reveal difference. Studying such affinity, she suggested, presented a challenge because it introduced the possibility that ethnographic research might lose its analytical capacity and become mere description. At the same time it presented an invaluable opportunity because it opened up new arenas to sociological and anthropological inquiry. Documents for instance, she argued, have the ability to be objects of study, analytical categories and a methodological orientation at the same time and the ethnographer's skill consists of keeping these aspects in view simultaneously (Riles, 2006b). This means looking *at* documents as objects of study in their own right whilst also looking *through* them in order to study something else, such as persons or relations. It is in the sense of Riles' answer to the challenge of familiarity posed by bureaucratic knowledge practices to those of social anthropology or sociology that we refer to the 'ethnographic' study of documents.

Riles' introduction to a recent edited volume outlines a programme of work and sets the scene for a selection of stimulating papers that demonstrate the importance of approaching, interrogating and ana- lysing documents ethnographically (Riles, 2006a). By directing the reader's attention to diverse documentary practices and local mean- ings, this collection serves as a reminder that the study of artefacts has so far focused on documents' strategic or instrumental character, thereby missing other aspects, such as their aesthetic dimensions (Reed, 2006). Paying attention to aspects other than artefacts' dis- ciplinary characteristics is rather novel for the study of inquest files. This is because the work of Michel Foucault has been so influential in the field since Lindsay Prior's pioneering studies on the organisation of death through the office of the coroner and the institution of the mortuary (Prior, 1985; Prior, 1987).

For Prior, the ordering of death was an extension of the discourse and technologies of modern biomedicine. In the case of the coroner, he asserted that what their profession claims to be a neutral – because technocratic and medicalised – language is actually a symbol of power as well as the instrument through which such power to observe, inves- tigate and explain is wielded (Prior, 1985). By citing death within a medical framework, Prior argued, it became possible to divide all deaths into either natural ones – those situated in a world of disease – or unnatural ones which could only be accounted for by chance. The categories have in common that they allow for the excision of human agency by situating death in a realm outside human control and disconnecting it from the sphere of the social, thereby permitting the inquest to focus on the medical and technological aspects of death investigation. Prior's study and his emphasis on the language of bureaucratic objectivity as a mark of power, struck a chord with us, and his insight that by medicalising certain kinds of death, death itself appears to be controllable, is a point that is germane to any attempt to understand the link between suicide and mental illness. Yet, based on our material, a more complex and contradictory relationship between the language of the inquest and power, knowledge and identities emerges. First, Prior seems to assume that the medicalisation of death is always oppressive because it denies human agency (Prior, 1985). However, the ethnographic work of Josef Dumit has shown that, in the case of schizophrenia, the presence of a biomedical diagnosis was welcomed by the families of schizophrenics, because it allowed them to challenge aetiologies that identified social – especially familial – relationships as the illness's cause (Dumit, 1997). We also found examples of bereaved families actively embracing diagnoses of mental illness in suicide cases. Perhaps the connections between biomedicine, mental health and identities warrant more careful consideration. Secondly, our research showed that human agency remained very much discernible in the files. Hence, we argue that what made the inquest files so fascinating was not that they were devoid of human agency, but rather that they presented an opportunity to study the ways in which different actors' agency was transformed. Finally, while disciplinary power in the Foucauldian sense certainly plays an important role in the management of death, including the inquest, we fear that too strong a focus on its totalising aspects ignores some evidence to the contrary. Our intention here is to draw out the distinctly human practices and concerns of some of the key agents involved in the creation of the suicide file: medical scientists, physicians, witnesses, and the deceased.

Central to these concerns is morality. The moral dimension of suicide discourse has been observed in studies of newspaper reports (Coyle and MacWhannell, 2002), young people (Fullager, 2003), and bereaved families (Owens *et al.*, 2008). The negotiation of morality and responsibility is central to how people make sense of suicidal behaviour, yet in the context of the inquest morality is bracketed out. This is because inquests are envisaged and enacted as fact-finding inquiries. The purpose of an inquest is to establish the identity of the deceased person and how, when, and where they died. It is not to establish who was responsible for the death, and coroners take great care to ensure that this point is understood by the interested persons and by anyone attending an inquest hearing.[2] As part of their duty to prevent further

---

[2]Properly interested persons are the only ones allowed to examine witnesses and inspect the file at the inquest, other than the coroner. According to the Coroners Rules (1984) properly interested persons are defined as next of kin as well as those benefitting from any insurance policy of the deceased person, insurers, anyone whose actions or omissions may have caused or contributed to the death, inspectors and the chief of police, representatives of any of the preceding groups, and anyone else deemed a properly interested person by the coroner.

deaths, coroners can make recommendations, but the inquest itself will only establish lines of causality. Questions of guilt have to be addressed by a separate court trial. They are not discussed as part of the inquest. This does not mean that concerns about morality are absent in the inquiry, only that they are not part of the official framing of the inquest. In addition, as far as this chapter is concerned we will not be focusing on the rights or wrongs of individual suicides but on the ways in which identities become visible in the inquest case files.

Reports by medical scientists, medical specialists and physicians

The coroner would ask for reports from medico-scientific professionals to establish if there had been any indications that the death under investigation may have been a suicide. GPs and psychiatrists were not the only medico-scientific experts present in the file. In fact their reports were rarer than those of pathologists and toxicologists whose analyses could be found in virtually all the files.[3] However, the latter had encountered the deceased only as a corpse. While corpses are ambiguous entities – no longer living, breathing human beings, but neither ordinary objects – they are nonetheless more easily separated from their social relations (Joralemon, 1995; Howarth, 1996; Richardson, 2000; Scheper-Hughes, 1992). In contrast, GPs and psychiatrists had known what was now 'the deceased' as 'the patient', that is when he or she was still alive and self-evidently entangled in relationships. Hence, their reports exposed the tensions surrounding the act of the suicide. Thus there existed a key distinction between those health professionals who knew the deceased person when they were alive and those who only encountered them as a corpse.

Reports on the deceased person as corpse

Berg and Bowker (1997) have suggested that the greater the extent to which a professional's report is prescribed, the lower is his or her status. They based this conclusion on their analysis of the files of cancer

---

[3]In England and Wales post-mortems were conducted in 94 per cent of deaths where an inquest took place (Allen, 2005).

patients. These files contained temperature lists and flowcharts for the nurses to record blood pressure, pulse, temperature, medication, and other measurements which were followed by the order form on which physicians would write down any diagnostic steps and changes in treatment for nursing staff to execute (Berg and Bowker, 1997). The physician's progress report came next. It was constituted by a pre-structured form documenting the patient's medical history up to the date of admission, which was succeeded by many unstructured pages of daily notes. Finally, there were computer printouts from laboratory information systems, results from bacteriological tests and X-rays, and letters written about the patient. In their totality, the different documents constituted and rearranged the cancer patient's body.

The documents that created the patient file offered insights into the hierarchy of medical work. Berg and Bowker identified important differences in terms of what individual medical professionals were allowed to contribute to the file which mapped onto the clinic's organisational hierarchy. The extremes were represented by the differences between the physician's progress notes which were unstructured and allowed their named authors to create their own narratives and the nurses' records which restricted their input to measurements and the ticking of boxes. In between these poles resided the broadly structured accounts of the clinical specialists, and the increasingly tightly organised notes of bacteriologists and radiographers (Berg and Bowker, 1997). Hence, the patient file became simultaneously the repository of and an active agent in the creation of professional hierarchies.

In the context of the inquest, pathologists tended to use standardised forms. In fact, the Coroners Rules 1984 even provide a pro-forma of a post-mortem report (Dorries, 2004). Yet, considering these reports in isolation can invite the wrong conclusions, because it overlooks the pathologist's role during the inquest and especially during the public hearing that concludes the coroner's investigation. The purpose of the post-mortem examination of the diseased person's body is to establish the medical causes of death, a process that unlike many other elements of the inquest, takes the wider circumstances of the death into account only cursorily.

The post-mortem reports in the files replicated the pathologist's progress in his or her examination of the corpse and began with a brief summary of the circumstances under which the death occurred, including the estimated time of death, as well as identifying details of the deceased person. They then proceeded to note external features before entering the body. External examination would establish the condition, gender, and state of care or neglect of the body, as well as noting outward signs of injuries, fresh and old scars, fresh evidence of medical interventions, or identifying features such as tattoos. Then, the pathologist would direct his or her attention inwards, investigating the body's systems, including its organs. At each step, he or she would note evidence of injuries or any other signs of diseases or abnormalities indicating a potential cause of death. Signs of trauma, such as haematomas of the brain, or broken bones were also reported.

The post-mortem reports' exclusive focus on the materiality of the body resulted in an explanation of death that recognised only intention-less natural processes. It was precisely the pathologist's tightly circumscribed role that lent his or her report authority in the context of an inquiry that did not address questions of culpability. The other reason pathologists could speak from an influential position of near objectivity was because they were not implicated in the death and had never met the deceased person while they were still alive. While inquests, as judicial procedures do not inquire into who caused the death, the question of responsibility remains salient to those giving evidence. However, the ways they engaged with this tension differed. While lay witnesses tended to stress their lack of awareness of the deceased person's intentions, GPs, psychiatrists and other medical professionals who had met the deceased person as their patient, emphasised those aspects of their treatment that were empirically-based, well-documented, and unequivocal.

Reports on the deceased person as patient

For the purpose of the inquest, the manner of death, previous suicide attempts, a history of depression and mental illness, especially recent or acute episodes, could all support the coroner in his or her decision to return a verdict of suicide. However, we argue that the documents created by the deceased person's physicians in response to the coroner's request were not only about establishing the deceased's intention to take his or her life, but were also about the creation of different identities. We will be using the statements written by GPs and psychiatrists to draw out two aspects in particular – the identity of the treating physician as a medical expert and the identity of the deceased as patient – to show how they were connected to the search for a causative agent.

The statements provided by GPs and psychiatrists were not organised according to an externally imposed structure, but followed an inherent order that responded to the questions of how long the physician had known the patient, why they had come to see them, what they had been treated for, drugs prescribed and interventions ordered, and whether these had been successful or not. These documents were not mere copies of accumulated medical records, but were purposive because they had been written retrospectively and on request of the coroner. This meant not only that they concentrated on any indications that the deceased had intended to take his or her life, but they also gave evidence of the treatment that the deceased had received, as well as asserting that this treatment had been appropriate under the circumstances. These accounts focused on the medical and technical aspects of therapeutic interventions and were informed by a conception of the mind as an organ that was primarily responsive to pharmaceutical intervention.

Hence, the reports' emphasis lay on treating the patients' symptoms with suitable drugs, including anti-depressants and other forms of psychiatric medication as illustrated by the documents written about the deceased David (Case 67) and Katherine (Case 86). The report by David's GP recounted in considerable detail how he had prescribed four different anti-depressants during the last month before his patient's death. In each case, it also stated the motives David had given for stopping a particular drug. Two reasons mentioned in the GP's letter were that David felt one drug was not working and that another had made him feel unwell. The document also recounted how the GP had reminded his patient that it was not the drugs that were causing his – David's – problems. Whereas David saw the medication and by implication the GP's treatment as the issue, the GP pointed the finger at the illness, which could be cured by medical intervention, provided the correct drug was found, and the patient was compliant. In the case of Katherine, identifying a reason for what amounted essentially to failed treatment – because the patient had died, rather than recovered – was more controversial because no diagnosis had been made and the GP situated responsibility for the death largely with the patient. Her GP stated in his letter that Katherine had not suffered from any psychotic illness and that her multiple issues were due to 'personality problems rather than other active disease'. He continued by remarking on the interactions between Katherine's 'psychological/psychiatric problems and her somatic symptoms' and concluded by expressing his regrets at being unable to provide the coroner with a more precise diagnosis.

Modern biomedicine proceeds by separating out causes (Foucault, 1994 [1973]), but the report of Katherine's GP showed the difficulties medical practitioners were confronted with when trying to disentangle the different causes they had identified. Here, 'the social' or 'personal' became a blanket concept for those aspects of the patient's life that were not under specialist control and where responsibility lay with the patient as a person rather than with his or her physical body or biologically-situated mind. This focus on agents amenable to medical intervention also opened up the possibility that failure of such interventions lay with the patient, rather than with the treatments. While Katherine's physician refrained from naming the patient as the reason why medical intervention had failed, preferring instead to evoke unspecified interactions between different agents, that included Katherine but were not restricted to her, Richard's psychiatrist was more explicit.

Richard (Case 100), who hanged himself, had been under psychiatric care to help him cope with post-traumatic stress disorder and depression. In his report, the psychiatrist identified non-compliance with the medication, an unwillingness to engage with different professionals, and a refusal of other treatment options as the impetus for Richard's suicide. Although the report mentions in passing that Richard had lost his job, had to cope with several deaths in the family, and 'other social circumstances' and recognises them as contributing to his depression becoming 'somewhat resistant to treatment', these factors are not further investigated and treated as of lesser importance than Richard's reluctance to comply with his treatment regime. And yet, the 'social', in the shape of showing that Richard was more than a non-compliant patient, leached into the file; in this instance through unexpected and unpredictable synergies between the psychiatrist's assessment and the witness statements.

In his report, the psychiatrist had remarked that Richard's wife supported her husband's decisions. But in the file, the psychiatrist's professional distance regarding his patient clashed to shocking effect with the intimacy and physicality of the statement that Richard's wife made. She told of how her husband had looked and felt when she cut him down and how she stayed with him, hugging and kissing him. Her suffering was confirmed by the police officer arriving at the scene who described her as 'very distraught, she was crying uncontrollably and refused to leave her husband'.

From the coroner's point of view these different aspects of Richard, the person, were relevant only insofar as they related to the purpose of the inquest. Yet, in the context of an ethnographic study of the inquest files, they illustrated how professional expertise and bureaucratic technology combined in the files to define certain relationships, and even certain aspects of relationships, as more relevant than others. Approaching the files ethnographically means that a very different account of Richard's life and death becomes possible: one that restores complexity, multi-dimensionality and contradictions to people's lives which the inquest itself aims to reduce in order to answer the questions of how someone died and whether they intended to.

The medical professionals' reports in the file created certain aspects of the person of the deceased. They were expressive of a modern medico-scientific epistemology that aimed to separate human states into distinct illnesses that were due to well-defined causes. In the case of GPs and psychiatrists, a focus on physically situated illnesses that could be treated by primarily pharmaceutical interventions was also discernible. Furthermore, for those medical professionals who had encountered the deceased as patient rather than as corpse, the need arose to demonstrate that they had acted appropriately and that their patient's death had been unpredictable and unavoidable. In doing so, the medical professionals created a very normative identity of the deceased as a patient, with the implication that their agency should be restricted to following the advice of the treating specialist. Yet, in the file medical reports commingled with other documents, such as witness statements that had the potential to show the deceased in a very different light.

Witness statements

The witness statements in the inquest files had been taken by police officers from those present at the scene of death, those who had been in contact with the deceased before his or her death, and those who had been close to him or her. Their objective was to report observations, but not opinions. The statements were originally recorded by hand on standard police forms, which were later trans-ferred into word-processed documents. They gave the name, age, and contact details of the witness, as well as the relationship in which the witness stood to the deceased. The remainder of the ori-ginal form was lined, but otherwise unstructured, therefore allowing the witnesses to produce their own narrative of the event and give an account of what they had observed or experienced first-hand.

While statement takers aimed to document the narrative in the witnesses' own words, such statements were not verbatim records of the interview. Rather, the events recounted in them had been con-secutively ordered and the narrative itself had been shaped by the need to be concise and to the point. In order to achieve this aim, statements were drafted first by a police officer using institutional conventions of language and content. These documents' hybrid pro-duction process and the need to fulfil institutional and legal require-ments, lent the accounts a shared appearance. Such efforts to direct witnesses' agency did not, however, conceal each statement's unique character or the immediate impact of the event on the statement giver. Compared to the reports by medical professionals, witness statements tended to display a greater degree of involvement of their authors with the deceased. Officially, witness statements were about the deceased, but unlike medical professionals, witnesses were often inextricably embroiled with the person whose death constituted the subject of the inquest.

Witnesses tended to disassociate themselves from the death and its causes not only because it implicated them, but also because they were shocked by its violence. Such trauma could express itself in different ways. It could be very explicit, as in the case of the woman who had tried to dissuade her neighbour to jump off a bridge (Case 37), but it might not always be immediate. For instance it was not until she had returned home that a woman who found the body of a young man was 'hit by the enormity of it all' (Case 45). Hence, irrespective of whether their distress was caused by their entangle-ment in the circumstances leading up to the death or in the viol-ence of witnessing, unless they were police officers or members of the emergency services on duty, witnesses lacked professional distance to protect themselves when confronted with death. Because of the way the identities of the deceased and the witnesses were entangled, testimonies regarding the former could only be generated in relation to the latter.

Witnesses in suicide cases were a motley assortment and included the very close, such as kin, as well as those whose only connection with the deceased person was the death itself. However, the witnesses tended to be united in their unfamiliarity with death and in facing it without the relative shelter provided by professionalism. While some of the witnesses avoided a close encounter with death, instead calling on other bystanders, the emergency services or the police to approach the body, others rushed to the scene. Accounts of the latter cases in particular – where the witnesses had handled the body – were often distinguished by the minute details recounted. The memory of how the deceased had looked and felt, the kind of aids they had used to kill themselves, and how the witnesses had tried to save their lives, lent these statements a particular clarity and almost a cinematic quality which could be distressing for researchers reading them (Fincham *et al.*, 2008). The witnesses' confrontation with death could elicit powerful reactions and intense emotions that were sometimes discernible from the statement. In some cases, the witnesses' distress was implicit in the document's history as when there were two witness statements by the same person in the file. The first would be incoherent or it would be incomplete, for instance closing with a remark by the statement taker that the interview had been postponed because the witness was too distraught to continue. At other times, a statement dating from several days after the discovery of the death suggested that the witness had needed time to calm down. Another way to learn how the encounter with death had affected a witness was through the accounts of other witnesses. For instance, the police officer at the scene described the father who had discovered his son's body and was now cradling him in his arms as 'hysterical with grief' and repeating over and over again: 'He's my son, my only son'. At other times, the effect the death had on the witnesses was explicitly acknowledged in the statement, as in the excerpt above from Case 37.

For those witnesses who had known the deceased before their death, making a statement always implicated them. On the one hand this was because their own identity was intertwined with the deceased and on the other, because they had to re-evaluate their past in the light of the death. In addition, as witnesses in the inquest their role was to close the gaps in the account left by the deceased. In other words they were called on to provide testimony for their own actions, but also as representatives of the dead. The inquest is non-adversarial and not concerned with guilt, and suicide is not a criminal offence. Yet the inquest process remains thoroughly entangled with the criminal and legal system (Davis *et al.*, 2002; Biddle, 2003). Considered in conjunction with the moral desire to have acted beyond reproach, it is not surprising that the witnesses tried to present their own conduct as favourably as possible in this public inquiry. We are not suggesting that the witnesses' performance was entirely under their control. Given the entanglement of their own identity with the deceased person, the shock of the death, and the unfamiliar and formal coronial system, their ability to exercise such control was limited, even if we assume that they possessed an awareness of what would be needed for such a performance to be successful (Goffman, 1959). Nonetheless there was some evidence in the files suggesting that witnesses were trying.

Not surprisingly though, the results tended to be mixed. In one case, a mother asserted that she had no idea why her son had taken his life as he was generally in good health. The only exception had been two hospitalisations. The first was for an overdose and the second had been an incident involving the mother and a glass that had smashed next to the son's head, making the reader wonder if the mother had actually thrown it at him. The suspicion that the young man's life had been more chaotic than his mother's statement suggested was corroborated by other documents in the files. Similarly, the girlfriend of another young man who had taken his life pointed out that he had had significant debts and had recently been made redundant from his job, though none of these details had been mentioned by the deceased's family. The statements by family members instead highlighted that the young man and his girlfriend had had a stormy relationship that was frequently 'on-off'. The two examples illustrate again how the documents in the file acted together to generate different and often contradictory aspects of the deceased, but they also offer an insight into how the identities of the witnesses and the deceased person are intertwined.

The most poignant illustrations of this point occurred in cases where a key relationship between the deceased and his or her partner was ending or had recently done so. The letter to the coroner of the long-standing partner of a young man, Stuart, who killed himself, made the complicated emotional mix that the bereaved as witnesses were struggling with rather explicit. The couple had been together since they had met at university more than six years before. For the last three years she had been working away, returning only on the weekend. This had lead the young woman 'to question her long-term position' regarding the relationship, culminating in her packing her possessions and Stuart helping her do so after they had decided together – so she felt – to break up. In her letter she referred to herself as Stuart's partner and requested a change in the wording of her original statement. The reason for a recent weekend spent apart had not been 'to think things through' she insisted, but to celebrate the birthday of an elderly relative. She also listed a number of other actions that suggested to her that Stuart could not have intended to take his life and ended her letter by contesting her witness statement to the police because she felt it had been written with 'a slant towards suicide' and she found it difficult to reconcile such a possibility with her memory of the 'intelligent and strong willed individual' she had known Stuart as (Case 46).

In their statements the witnesses were working through their connections with the dead as well as with the living and in the process were generating themselves, the deceased and others living as persons. While they were maintaining connections with the deceased they also reassessed them in light of the death. This could mean that the bereaved attempted to extricate themselves from relationships by de-emphasising their own entanglement with the act, as in the case of the young woman above. They may also do so by arguing that the suicide could not have been foreseen ('he seemed happy'), even when other evidence suggested otherwise, or they may make reference to mental illness as a causal factor. As a result, the bereaved – like the physicians and as we will see, the deceased – tried to transfer the reasons for the suicide into a sphere outside their area of responsibility and control. In the case of medical professionals, this external realm included 'the social', but the witnesses and the deceased transferred the act into the sphere of naturally, rather than socially, occurring incidents and events; that is, events and actions that were somehow unavoidable (as opposed to those that could potentially have resulted in a different outcome). However, not only could such sequestration never be total, but the witnesses' entanglement with the deceased as persons, as well as their role as witnesses in the inquest process, including standing for the deceased and lacking a protective professional persona to fall back on, made their situations much more ambiguous and difficult to bear. Hence the tensions that were generated by the questions about the causes of the suicide continued. As researchers we only have the inquest records to go by and while these can produce fascinating and unexpected insights, we cannot know to what extent the witnesses' accounts of their role in the death were 'true'. This is not a methodological weakness, because from a dual paradigms perspective, alongside the question of 'truth' about suicide we have to ask what we can learn from the files about the complex, contradictory and often harrowing experience of having been bereaved by suicide and finding oneself a witness in an inquest.

Suicide notes

The final category of documents we will turn to are the suicide notes that were present in almost half of our sample. In the following chapter we will examine more closely individual suicide notes to investigate issues of agency, apology and relationality. Here we are concerned only with what the notes contributed to the inquest files and the identities they created. Suicide notes are important in the inquest, because they supply evidence of the deceased person's intent to take his or her life and thereby help to support a verdict of suicide. They vary greatly in their form and content and are the only documents in the file that have been written by the hand of the deceased. Coroners should usually release the note to the original addressee as soon as possible after the inquest, although they may retain a photocopy of it. Not having a suicide note is considered to interfere with the grieving process (Biddle, 2003).

Suicides notes in inquest files are special, because only a fraction of people taking their life will leave a note, with figures ranging from 18 to 37 per cent (see next chapter). But suicide notes are remarkable in other ways, too. For a start, they are the only document that has been written by the deceased, rather than about him or her and like a signature they come to stand for the person who wrote them.

They are also the only documents in the file that had been produced before the deceased died. Because they were created before the inquest was opened, they were exempt from the requirements of having to give account at an official investigation. And yet, similarly to lay witnesses statements they were trying to minimise the extent to which individual agency played a role in the death.

Irrespective of their length, their eloquence, or the sentiments they expressed, the notes shared the basic premise that the only course of action available to their authors was to take their own life. They had been forced into a situation where they had been 'in pain for too long now and [...] can't take no more', where 'enough is enough', and where '[t]here was no other way' (Jacobs, 1967). At the same time, they had been brought to this realisation, by circumstances lying outside their control. Thus, the person about to commit suicide constructed a scenario where forces outside their command were acting on them. Under these circumstances, taking one's life became an act of self-assertion, a way to exert power over forces otherwise too powerful to control. Yet such an act also implied the exclusion of other people, because the knowledge on which the decision to end his or her life was based could only be possessed by the person about to die.

At the same time, the notes were an attempt by the deceased to influence the future, an act that required some form of connection with the living. The following chapter analyses more closely how suicide notes were intended to exert agency after the death of their author. At this point it suffices to say that in the context of the file, the different identities of deceased person, such as son and spouse, could diverge from those created by other documents accumulated during the course of the inquest. This can be illustrated by the man who wrote one note to his mother in which he apologised for his act, and another note to his wife in which he congratulated her on winning; or by the case of Mark, in the previous chapter, who evoked the negative impact his death would have on the development of the son he had had with an ex-partner, threatening that his memory would always stay with her, and with it her liability for his death. Admittedly, no guarantees existed that such evocations would become reality, and this also applied to the instructions to the bereaved not to be sad about the death, but instead to get on with their lives. An example of how incapable the deceased were of affecting the reception of their suicide notes concerned a young man who had mentioned feelings of loneliness and emptiness as causes for the act, while his file contained a memo inquiring about the state of an investigation regarding sexual offences the deceased had been accused of in an adjacent jurisdiction. Thus, similarly to the witness statements, in the file the self-presentation of the authors often encountered other documents that cast doubt over the truthfulness and completeness of their explanations. In summary, the suicide notes in the files illustrated that not only can existing identities persist, but also new ones can be created.

Conclusion

At the beginning of this chapter we mentioned the argument that identities can potentially be maintained in death. Our study of inquest files supports this argument to some extent. An example of this process is the suicide notes, as attempts by the deceased to exert agency from beyond the grave. We can also establish that such attempts to influence their legacy are hampered by the deceased person no longer possessing control over a functioning physical body which made it impossible to counteract the unpredictable synergies created by the different documents that constitute the inquest file. Without an ability to act, the deceased could not confront any challenges to their version of what has happened and why, unless the living responded on the deceased's behalf, an effect the suicide notes aim to achieve.

We also found that the dead could possess different identities in the course of an inquest, such as those of patient, son, and spouse or partner. They could equally acquire new ones such as being a victim of uncontrollable circumstances. Furthermore, the files showed that the identities of the deceased – like those of the living – could be contradictory, as in the conflicting demands of patient and spouse. However, our material equally demonstrated that while relational social identities continued after death, there was evidence of all the actors in the files minimising their ability to influence the course of action. This included medical professionals, who argued that the act was due to factors outside their control, and witnesses close to the deceased who tended to insist that the death could not possibly have been foreseen. Finally, the deceased themselves asserted that they had no choice but to commit suicide. In other words, everyone in the file was concerned with playing down their own agency and demonstrating that they themselves were not at fault. There is a paradoxical finding here insofar as agency is visible within these various documents, but their 'intention' is very much about the denial of agency.

For the social anthropologist Alfred Gell (1998), intention is what distinguishes primary agency from secondary agency. Objects, such as landmines, or documents might have agency, insofar as they make things happen. What they lack is the ability to act intentionally. Only human beings, Gell posits, can have such primary agency, which distinguishes them from the secondary agency of objects. Yet, there are situations in which the primary agency of humans has been compromised, and in fact, many social institutions, such as the army, are designed to manage human agency in this way. The transformation of primary into secondary agency is central to inquests, insofar as they are intended and enacted to dissipate the consequences of identifiable individual actions in favour of intention-less 'natural' processes (Langer, 2010). The suicide verdict seems at first exceptional here as evidence of death being the intended outcome of an action is a prerequisite for it. As we have seen in the initial discussion of suicide notes, this interpretation is largely resisted by the deceased who portray their actions as impermeable to personal choice. This neglect of primary agency, and the responsibility it implies, occurred in spite of inquests not being about the apportionment of blame and we have demonstrated that concerns about culpability remained latent, suggesting a shared cultural concern with situating suicide outside the sphere of human agency.

By taking an ethnographic approach to the study of documents, we have been able to show how identities manifest themselves in the files, as well as drawing attention to the ways in which different actors in the suicide files were engaged in a process of separating out what could be avoided from what was unavoidable or, to put this differently, identifying those aspects over which they had a degree of influence in contrast to those over which they had none. While for physicians the unavoidable was largely part of the social domain, for witnesses it was the natural domain, such as the presence of mental illness, which was beyond their reach. Because of these different emphases, the statements of medical professionals and witnesses were frequently at odds. The documents had in common, though, a concern with minimising their authors' association with potential motives for the suicide. Thus, the study of inquest files of suicide also provided an opportunity to analyse the ways in which culturally specific notions of relationships and of personhood infused the bureaucratic processes of the coroner's investigation.

5
Suicide Notes as Social Documents

In this chapter our focus is on the suicide notes that nearly half of the files contained. In keeping with the sociological autopsy approach we treat the notes not as straightforward indicators of mental illness, but as culturally-specific artefacts that bring into relief the role of social relationships in instances of suicide. We will approach the notes as a means of connection, as well as drawing attention to their content, structure and material form. In particular we ask how the use of suicide notes as an apology and as a claim to victimhood can help to establish a relationship where none existed previously or to re-establish one that had been severed. We suggest that this usually happens with a sense towards improving the deceased person's chances of having their final wishes heeded. Hence this chapter is also an exploration of agency from beyond the grave.

Psychiatry and psychology are the disciplines that have been most concerned with the study of suicide and its prevention and given the methodological basis of these disciplines, it is not surprising that until recently suicide notes have largely been studied with the help of quantitative methods and with an eye towards the discovery of generalisable rules. This scientific epistemology has been used exhaustively to study suicide notes, for instance to establish differences between genuine and faked notes (Black, 1993; Jones and Bennell, 2007), between attempters and completers (Leenaars et al., 1992; Handelman and Lester, 2007) or between different nationalities (Zonda, 1999; Wong et al., 2009; O'Connor and Leenaars, 2004; Girdhar et al., 2004; Leenaars et al., 2010). In addition suicide notes have been studied by gender (Canetto and Lester, 2002), occupational group (Aggarwal, 2008), across the life-course (Salib, Cawley and Healy, 2002; Leenaars, 2003) and to test different hypotheses, such as psychological theories of suicide (e.g. Schneidman and Farberow, 1957; Leenaars, 1988). Yet such comprehensive investigation did not translate into unequivocal answers, with some authors concluding that suicide notes provided only limited insight into the causes of suicide (O'Donnell *et al.*, 1993) and even Edwin Schneidman, who pioneered suicidology and the study of suicide notes, reflected in later life that the notes may not be the royal road to understanding suicide that he had once thought and that they were frequently banal and dull (quoted in Sanger and McCarthy Veach, 2008: 354).

However, there is some suggestion that the lacklustre findings gained from the study of suicide notes so far may be less of a reflection of the notes themselves and their authors, than evidence of methodological weaknesses, such as studies that have been limited to a small selection of samples or comprising only a handful of cases. Furthermore, most studies of suicide notes have been restricted to the notes themselves, thereby excluding potentially important contextual data. Such a limitation does not apply to psychological autopsies, a method that allows researchers to take into account the diverse factors shaping lives ending in suicide, but here the note becomes only one amongst a multitude of sources. Equally problematic has been that comparisons between groups, one of the mainstay of research on suicide notes, has been based on ostensibly 'natural' categories that neglect heterogeneity within groups, such as in terms of the differences between people who happen to live – or rather die – in the same country, or they have focused on biologically-grounded or normatively conceptualised categories such as 'men' or 'women' (for a critique, Scourfield, 2005). Most glaring, however, has been the virtual exclusion of qualitative research (Hjelmeland and Knizek, 2010).

Until recently, the only notable exceptions have been papers by Jacobs (1967) and by Utriainen and Honkasalo (1996), the former being a phenomenological study of 112 suicide notes from the Los Angeles area, the latter a feminist semiotic analysis of suicide notes by Finnish women. Yet the arrival of a number of new studies offers evidence of much needed novel impulses being introduced into the field (McClelland *et al.*, 2000; Knizek and Hjelmeland, 2007; Sanger and McCarthy Veach, 2008). McClelland *et al.* (2000) took a discursive approach to the study of 172 suicide notes, written by

120 authors. They studied the notes not in order to uncover any underlying psychological reasons, but to investigate the management of blame. As the authors correctly argue, this requires that suicides notes are seen not as straightforward representation of the state of the mind of the deceased person before they died, but rather as a form of communication between those about to take their lives and those they leave behind. The authors state that matters relating to blame featured in 87 per cent of their sample. Such blame is either directed at self or less often at others, yet is treated in different ways. The issue of self-blame is raised because the person about to die wants to deny or mitigate it, and while some constructions of other-blame are concerned with mitigation, other intend to point the finger.

McClelland *et al.*'s paper is a refreshing departure from the often rather formulaic and simplistic approaches to the study of suicide notes that have dominated the field for so long. Yet we are concerned that the focus on blame can be analytically problematic, because it distracts from the fact that suicide notes are inherently conflicted and conflicting, as these authors recognise when they point out that self-blame and other-blame can be closely entangled (McClelland *et al.*, 2000). Having said this, we agree that blame, its management and associated themes of responsibility and agency, play a major role in suicide notes, including in our sample. In fact, it could not be otherwise, as this reflects how suicide is often framed in common discourse and, as we will demonstrate, those taking their lives do not act outside culture.

Instead of questions of culpability, we will concentrate in this chapter on agency and relationships. As mentioned previously, relationships make persons. Hence being able to establish a link with the living even after death, through a suicide note, is about something more fundamental than the negotiation of blame. Rather, such a relationship enables the continuation of the deceased person as a person. Undoubtedly, they have become a different kind of person, yet through the note they have nonetheless managed to extend their existence.

In our view it is their recognition of the centrality of relationships that gives Sanger and McCarthy Veach's article (2008) its relevance. In their study of 138 suicide notes written between 1944 and 1968, they pay attention to the interpersonal nature of suicide and identify seven themes: instructions, positive relationships, explanations, relationship reconciliation/maintenance, concern for others, negative relationship, and acknowledging the end of a relationship. With regards to the current chapter, one of their most important findings is that positive relationships were more prevalent than negative ones, that many of the notes expressed concern for others, and that relationships contribute to suicide motives. We agree that many notes do indeed express gratitude and care for the bereaved, but we would caution against taking them as the whole story. In this case it is important that in addition to the notes we were able to draw on further contextual information generated during the inquest process. Unlike what might naively be assumed, from a sociological and anthropological point of view, such supplementary data do not necessarily clarify the emerging picture, but rather complicate it. Thus, case files act as a reminder of the contradictions often surrounding acts of suicide and demand recognition of the limits of our ability to know. Such an acceptance of the partiality of all knowledge regarding suicide can then become the starting point for further investigation. Furthermore, we feel that Sanger and McCarthy Veach did not quite follow through with their own argument about the centrality of connections in order to understand suicide, because if suicide notes are about interconnectedness, then death is not the end. Having said this, their paper represents a very promising new line of exploration in the study of suicide notes, as well as suicide and its prevention.

Probably the most ambitious of this recent series of qualitative studies of suicide notes is by Knizek and Hjelmeland (2007) who develop a sophisticated model of suicide notes as communication that combines semiotics with hermeneutics and conversation analysis. Pointing out the need for suicidology to establish a shared terminology they argue for the development of a new paradigm that is able to accommodate both qualitative and quantitative approaches and do justice to the complexity of its subject matter. They proceed by outlining a model that they consider to be both theory-based and able to analyse suicide notes as a form of communication. We welcome Knizek and Hjelmeland's intellectually stimulating and audacious initiative, because it introduces new ideas into the study of suicide notes. Specifically, we welcome the authors' championing of qualitative research as a suitable approach for the study of suicide. Furthermore, their interpretation of suicide notes as communication chimes with us, because it recognises the notes as social documents that connect, entangle, and to an extent create, different kinds of persons, rather than seeing them only as manifestations of mental illness. Despite these areas of connection, our agenda in this book is different from Knizek and Hjelmeland's. Our focus is not on developing a model to interpret suicide notes, but rather a methodology for studying lives that end in suicide. And we do not aim to develop an elaborated theory of suicidal behaviour but rather to make connections between our data and a wide range of theoretical reference points, which are more likely to have disciplinary origins in sociology, social anthropology or psychoanalysis than in semiotics. Our inquiry engages with persons and objects, rather than speech acts. At the core of this approach lies a concern with relationships that incorporates their material and embodied aspects, as well as their ability to call into question everyday certainties about distinctions such as self and other or life and death.

As we have shown in the preceding chapter, the identities of the living and the dead were inextricably intertwined, which gives us reason to disagree to an extent with Knizek and Hjelmeland's (2007) emphasis on interactions between actor and recipients. Although the inquest with its clearly defined roles encourages such an interpretation, close reading of the documents constituting the file suggested otherwise. Instead, it demonstrates how mixed up different identities were, especially in the case of witnesses and the deceased. To us, this points at relationships not simply existing between persons, but rather as being constitutive of them. In the preceding chapter we were concerned with the creation of identities and showed that in spite of the inquests being ostensibly concerned with clarification, in the files the identities of those affected by suicide were deeply entangled. Our approach in this chapter on suicide notes is similar in that it argues for the permeability of boundaries that are often seen as impenetrable. Rather than seeing death as the end, we show how suicide notes can be a means to continue or even to initiate relationships through which agency can be exerted.

Approaching suicide notes from a social science perspective

As previously mentioned, at the moment the study of suicide notes is largely the preserve of psychiatrists and psychologists, with some support by the humanities in the form of philosophy and communication theory. Such dominance raises the question whether the social sciences are suited to the study of suicide notes at all, let alone whether they can add anything substantial? We suggest that the answer to both questions is 'yes'. To begin with, our disciplines' emphasis on the social and cultural dimensions of the notes can offer valuable insights into suicidal lives, instead of mental pathology. We consider this a pertinent distinction regarding suicide notes, because as will become clear shortly, the people in our sample who had written the notes considered them to be important messages and wrote them with the intention to be understood. This is evident from the physical features of the suicides notes, but also from their structure and content. This means that while the notes are as individual as their authors, they are also, like their authors, part of a wider social and cultural context. In addition we consider the contribution of the social sciences to come from three areas of study in particular: documents, agency, and death. We have already illustrated in the preceding chapter how documents can affect identities in the context of the inquest process. Here we will predominantly focus on the latter two aspects but will be paying brief attention to the material features of suicide notes, too.

Forty-nine of the people in our sample had written suicide notes, though in one case the existence of this note was only mentioned, but neither did the artefact of the note find its way into the file nor did its content. These notes had a total of 94 addressees. Sometimes the authors wrote individual notes for each addressee, but they might also address different people in the same note, making categorisation more difficult. In terms of those who were mentioned in the notes 22 were former or present spouses or partners, 33 were family members and 39 of the notes were addressed to others. Notes in the last category included flat mates and work colleagues and people who may have played a role in the lead-up to the death. Most commonly however, the notes were directed at the emergency services, in particular the police, or were simply for 'whoever may find me'. Of the 33 notes to family members, two were addressed to family members in the wider sense, one to a nephew, one to the deceased person's mother-in-law and six were for siblings. Parents were the recipients of seven notes, of which one was addressed to both father and mother, four to the deceased person's mother and two to his or her father. Eight notes were blanket messages to the whole family and ten were specifically for the deceased person's children.

The overwhelming emotion expressed in the suicide notes was a sense of deep regret, which for instance was evident in the prominent place of apologies, which were often linked to expressions of gratitude. Inherent to the sense of regret in the notes was that nothing could prevent the suicide. Though the authors of the suicide notes rarely went into detail, the reasons were diverse. They included fear of incapacity and decrepitude, loneliness and the end of important relationships, as well as a sense of shame and generalised failure. The notes conveyed these feelings as facts, as if the writer had simply reached a point in their life at which suicide was the only choice available. It was a choice, but for the person about to die, it was also the only choice. Other emotions discernable were a sense of self-pity and also in some instances a sense of anger and aggression. Yet on the whole, the most common approach was to strive for a largely factual tone of voice in the suicide notes.

Not all suicide notes came to us in their original form, because from the point of view of the inquest their material appearance was insignificant. All that mattered was their content, namely whether the notes gave evidence of the deceased person's intention to die. This means that information about the physical appearance of the note was not always recorded, although police officers at the scene would confiscate any evidence of how the deceased had died, including tablet strips and notes. While we were not always able to examine the original note, we would usually be able to work with photo-copied or word-processed copies. Despite these limitations which were imposed on us by the purpose of the inquest, we were able to accumulate sufficient data to develop an idea of typical properties of suicide notes.

A surprising feature of those suicide notes whose physical appearance we know something about is that the vast majority were written on paper. We found no evidence of suicide notes having been sent by email and in only three instances had the deceased expressed his or her intention to die by text message. Given the way in which communication by text message has become part of the everyday fabric of relationships, this seems surprising. To illustrate, by July 2005, 66 per cent of adults in Great Britain had sent a text message and 68 per cent had received one (ONS, 2007). Figures by the Mobile Data

Association show a steep continual rise of text messages sent over the last decade, that so far has culminated in a daily average of 265 million text messages in 2009 (http://text.it/mediacentre). This means that in keeping with this trend the proportion of suicide notes via text message is likely to have risen since we completed data collection, even though text messaging is the preferred form of communication of the young, rather than the middle-aged and the old who constituted the majority in our sample.

Yet there may also have been other reasons for the rarity of suicide notes by text message. Commonly text messages are used for fairly casual communications and it is still considered bad form to send important information via this medium. This is especially true if the message is likely to affect the recipient negatively, for instance, if they are told of the end of a relationship, or the termination of their job. Keeping this in mind, the fact that of the 49 people who left suicide notes, only three had done so using text messages, suggests that these missives were considered significant and special. It also indicates that their authors had an awareness of their action affecting the recipients in a negative way. Furthermore, compared to paper, text messages are ephemeral and easily deleted, another reason, we think, why the traditional form of written communication dominated. It is certainly possible that the preference for old-fashioned paper over modern telecommunication was connected to the limitations of digital technology, such as length of messages. But while a couple of the suicide notes ran to nearly 1000 words, the average length was 126 words. Typically, the notes covered only a few lines, suggesting that other considerations played a role when people about to die decided on a medium for their final message.

Another reason to infer that their authors attach importance to the suicide notes comes from the actual material they are written on and from their physical appearance. Some of the notes had undoubtedly been written on the first piece of paper available. For instance, one note was written on the back of an amplifier instruction booklet, while another one was written on police incident paper, and a third on the back of a letter from social services. On the whole, though, the notes were written on ordinary notepads, recognisable by their lines and ripped out perforations, or more formally had been word-processed or used letter-headed paper. We also found evidence of the notes having been rewritten, in a few instances. Such signs of preparation and planning do not mean that the notes were free from indicators of agitation or distress. Some notes showed stains and blotches and others were full of spelling mistakes, random capitalisation and crossed out words. Nonetheless, the notes were meant to be understood and their authors were very much concerned to appear of sound mind:

> Yes, I have had some VODKA but am in control of myself.
> (Case 33)

In most of the notes, this desire to be taken seriously was not as explicit as in the above quotation and had to be inferred from their appearance and structure. This can be illustrated by the notes left by a young man who took his life because he was convinced that this would delay the repossession of the parental home. He left behind five neatly typed letters: to his brother, to trusted friends, to his team leader at work and to a colleague explaining in remarkable detail and entirely lucidly what they needed to do for his plan to succeed. At the same time, he did not consider that the plan itself may be 'mad'. The care and control displayed in these suicide notes suggests that even where there were indications of mental health problems, the person about to take his or her life wanted to be understood. Being understood is the precondition to ensuring that the notes had an effect. In this case, the purpose of the suicide was to delay the repossession as to enable the bereaved family and friends to remove anything from the house. A more typical note would still be intended to have an effect, though one that was not as specific and required a lesser degree of organisation and coordination.

The inquest file did not record whether the young man's scheme was successful beyond leading to his death, but he certainly took every precaution to guarantee its success, including a performance of sanity. We cannot know whether the vodka drinker in Case 33 above was still *compos mentis*. What matters in relation to a social science approach to suicide notes is the authors' intention to be recognised as someone who is in full possession of their critical faculties. Whether they achieve this aim or not may remain moot, yet from a sociological or social anthropological point of view that is concerned with relationships, the suicide notes have to be taken at face value.

The above examples show that people who died of suicide were not outside 'normal' society and its conventions, at least not those who left behind notes. Rather they used existing conventions regarding written communication – such as appearing rational – to make their point about the inevitability of ending their lives. There is a further aspect that demonstrates that people about to take their lives operated within shared conventions, namely that their suicide notes had to be recognised as such in order to have made it into the inquest files. The suicide notes were found on the deceased person, at or near the place where the person had died, or where they had lived. In one instance, the note had been posted to the deceased person's bereaved parents. In addition to the site where the suicide note was found, it is also their appearance and structure that helps to identify what they are and that alerts police officers to retain them and hand them over to the coroner. In the coroner's court, the existence of a suicide note is in itself insufficient evidence for a verdict of suicide.

The claim that sociology and social anthropology can make a relevant contribution to the study of suicide, including suicide notes, is not solely based on acknowledging the fact of people taking their own life being a part of society. It is also rooted in the recognition that suicide notes create, repair and extend social relationships between people, across time, and between life and death. These connections were seen to have consequences. That is, they were the conduit through which effects – from requesting music to be played at the funeral, to shaping the memory of the deceased person, to affecting the suicide's impact on the bereaved – could be achieved. This means that in the definition of the social anthropologist Alfred Gell (1998), the notes possess agency, insofar as they cause events. This is possible because for Gell, agency is not restricted to physical actions, but also includes intentions. Yet importantly, only human beings can have intentions, leading Gell to distinguish between secondary agency – such as those of the notes – and primary agency – as of their authors. Having said this, in the notes their authors' primary agency is conspicuously muted. This we suggest is because intention also introduces the possibility of culpability.

Apologies in suicide notes as connection

Two thirds of the suicide notes we studied contained an apology or a request for forgiveness for having taken their lives:

> Mum + Dad, I'm sorry I have done this to you I really am. (Case 40)

Such apologies were not limited to close kin or (ex-)partners, but also were made to friends and to those who might find the body:

> To the police, firstly may I say how sorry I am for all the hassle I have caused. And also sorry to the person who found me. (Case 7)

This raises the question that if the deceased person's death was as inescapable as he or she portrayed it in the suicide note then why the need to apologise? In other words, a valid apology can only be made by someone responsible for their actions. The answer is that apologies establish relationships which in turn are a precondition for efficacy of the suicide note. This is all the more important in the case of death, and suicide in particular, because it is commonly conceived as the end of all social connection. In our sample of suicide notes, only five talked about death as signifying the beginning of a different existence. Although views about how they would continue to exist after death were generally quite vague one theme was that it would allow them to move to a better place, either because they would be 'happy' there or because they hoped to 'be at peace now'. Hence, while not being explicit about what would await them after death, the writers were hoping for an improvement of their current situation and those who saw themselves still to be part of a network of social relationships were looking forward to being reunited with a loved one who had pre-deceased them or to welcoming their friends in the future. Some also imagined that their concern and love for their family and friends could still be experienced by the living even though they were now longer amongst them. Yet those who envisaged some form of continued existence and a reunion with friends and loved ones were in the minority. Most of the people who left behind suicide notes, did not mention anything about what would happen after death. In these notes, death was nothingness. In this they exemplified a modern Western view of life and death as polar opposites.

Unlike societies in other places where the dead, as a collectivity of ancestors, play a crucial role in the well-being of the living by regenerating life (Harris, 1982), or other times, such as medieval Europe where the dead could influence the extent of the dying person's time in purgatory, in modern Western societies the dead and the living inhabit separate worlds with no connection and no ability to affect the other (Howarth, 2007). Bloch and Parry suggest that suicide is – especially in Christian cultures – 'the supreme example of a "bad" death' because it lacks the potential for rebirth and regeneration' (1982: 16). Having said this, other research suggests that it is not so much suicide's absence of regenerative potential that marks it out as a 'bad' death, but rather that it contravenes aspects of what constitutes a 'good' death. For instance, 'good' deaths happen in old age, they are painless, occur in private and peaceful surroundings and with loved ones present, and the dying person is able to exercise a degree of control over their death (Bradbury, 1996). In contrast, the deceased people in our sample, while largely middle-aged, were mostly too young to be expected to die naturally, and the deaths themselves contravened conventions of the 'good' death because they happened in public and involved parks, railway lines, bridges, or tall buildings, or took place away from family and friends, or because they were sometimes violent or painful. However, Bradbury's final point about the importance of control in the 'good' death is potentially problematic because suicide means that the person died by their own volition and therefore should have possessed considerable control over the circumstances of their death. Yet reasoning in this way overlooks that from the point of view of the deceased person, their death was due to developments and events outside their control. Thus, because they are often distressing and challenge expectations of deaths and dying, common characteristics of suicides can intensify the feeling of disruption of social connections caused by death. For instance Wertheimer (1990) attests that the loss induced by suicide is experienced as a more intense feeling of bereavement than other forms of death.

Apologies not only have a role to play in notes to those who used to be close to the deceased person. They may also serve to establish a relationship where none existed prior to the death. In the notes, apologies where commonly followed by requests and exhortations, including ones addressed to emergency services personnel, police officers, or witnesses. For instance the notes requested that their authors would not be resuscitated, or that additional notes saved on the deceased person's mobile phone would be accessed, or asked that police ensure that objects and messages would reach their intended addressees and that the last wishes of the dying person would be executed in the specified way. After having apologised to the person who found him, and to the police, this man made the following request:

> With this letter there is a Dictaphone which I request goes to my MUM and also a letter which I would like hand delivered to [*this address*] this is [*ex-partner's*] friend's address but you will [*find*] her there. Please do not mention this letter to any of my family it will only hurt them more. One last thing, if anything from my body can be used to help somebody else, you have my permission.
> (Case 7)

Here, the apology helped to establish a relationship that could become a conduit for the deceased person's agency. The apology says 'we have something in common, whether you want it or not'. However, not only are the assumptions involved in making an apology a murky affair as Rapport (2009) writes, but there is also no way for the deceased person to ensure that their wishes will be fulfilled. For instance, we do not know whether the bereaved family were informed of the existence of other letters and what effect this had on them, nor can we be certain that the Dictaphone was indeed delivered to the deceased person's mother. This was the risk that the dying person had to take, but by including an apology in their request they hoped to increase his or her chances that it would be acted on.

Following Rapport, we propose that the presence and frequency of apologies in suicide notes is significant because an apology establishes a relationship, in this case between the writer and the recipient of a suicide note. He outlined two aspects of an apology: as a claim to knowledge and as a claim to responsibility. As a claim to knowledge, an apology professes to know of a situation that the speaker wishes had not occurred or that he or she knows the recipient wishes had not occurred. These claims are based on assumptions the speaker can never be certain of. As a claim to responsibility, an apology states that the speaker knows of a situation which the speaker or the group they wish to speak for have caused to happen. The two facets of apology converge in establishing a relationship (Rapport, 2009: 350–1, original emphasis):

> A claim to responsibility, one could say, is a claim to a relationship: both to the perpetrator (either myself or my fellow)

and to the sufferer. And a claim to knowledge (of something to be sorry about) is *also* a claim to a relationship.

In the context of suicide notes, as we have illustrated, this relationship between the person apologising and the one he or she apologises to cannot be taken for granted. This is not only because death is commonly imagined as the end of all relationships, but also because of differences in terms of quality or duration of the relationship that existed between the author of the note and the recipient before the suicide. Hence even where a relationship continued up to the death an apology was appropriate. Yet what about instances where author and recipient had never met? For example, notes addressed to the emergency services or to the unknown person who would find the body fall into this category. Finally, how are connections being established where a relationship had been terminated during the deceased person's lifetime, such as when a suicide note was addressed to a former partner? We describe in this book (see Chapter 7 in particular) how suicidal acts can follow relationship breakdown – i.e. the end of a committed intimate relationship. In our sample, in 14 cases, 11 men and three women, there was evidence of relationship breakdown and a suicide note had been written to a former partner. This is a small proportion and what follows can only be considered a cursory analysis. Connections are established firstly through apologies, secondly by mention of 'love', and thirdly by acknowledgement of the relationship in its absence. Sometimes different approaches are combined, as in the example below.

> [*Former partner's name*],
> I loved you truly. I just couldn't face life without you. I am so very sorry.
> I LOVE YOU.
> XXXXXXXXXX
> My life to grave my love for you. Look after the kids.
> XXX
> (Case 88)

Like an apology, the expression of 'love' is a claim to a relationship, whether the other person wants it or not, as are the children. And yet, it is the former partner's absence that made it impossible for the deceased person to carry on.

Finally, in the case of intimate relationship breakdown, relationships could be established by stressing that the ex-partner was not welcome, not even after death:

> One thing I would ask is you don't use your position as my next of kin to claim against my estate.
> (Case 43)

Here the separated wife is told to keep away and the relationship exists as an inversion. In other words, rather than acting as a conduit to make things happen, here the intention is in making sure that nothing happens, or least nothing involving the former spouse.

Following Rapport, we have suggested that apologies help to establish relationships, but he also identified two inherent qualities of apologies: a claim to knowledge and a claim to responsibility. We have shown how an apology acts as a claim to knowledge in the suicide: the author knows of something about to happen and he or she makes the assumption that their actions will cause pain and hurt in the recipient of the note. But what about an apology as a claim to responsibility (Rapport, 2009: 350)?

> As a claim to responsibility, an apology says that I know of a situation which I caused to happen or the group which I claim to speak for caused to happen. And again, I know you would wish it had not occurred. At least, I assume this because I certainly wish it had not occurred.

Now, some of the people who left behind suicide notes took responsibility for their actions.

> This is the first time in my life that I've ever felt so sure about something and I know I'm going to achieve what I set out to do.
> (Case 8)

But such bold statements asserting the deceased person's agency and the correctness of their decision were relatively rare. Usually, they were tempered by statements that show the person about to die is aware that their actions will have painful consequences for the bereaved, but that this cannot be helped and may even be for the best of all:

> I know I am doing an awful thing and you could really do with the support. Unfortunately I am unable to provide it.
> (Case 69)

In this case, the man who took his life had recently lost his job and feared the revelation of other inadequacies in his work, but other notes simply stated that the deceased had intended to take their lives all along and that nothing the living might have done would have changed their mind.

> I've been suicidal for over 4 years which is why I got so good at acting 'ok' and it's always been a case of 'when' rather than 'whether'. There's nothing that anyone could've said or done to change my mind so that's why I never talked to anyone about it: there wasn't any point (and would have made whoever I talked to feel guilty when I actually went ahead with it).
> (Case 70)

In this note, suicide is presented as a *fait accompli* and because it is a foregone conclusion there is no need for an explanation. This absence of a justification of 'why' the person has to die, is quite striking in the notes. The suicide becomes a fact of life (or rather death) that is unavoidable and inescapable, comparable to an incurable illness that strikes randomly and for which the question 'why me?' becomes meaningless.

What the notes intend to accomplish

While suicide notes might be assumed to contain rather dramatic content, in fact they often seem quite mundane. They appear so because they make visible the everyday activity of relationship creation and maintenance that constitutes human beings as persons. The notes are social documents that use other persons and objects to extend the deceased person beyond death by affecting the way the bereaved will remember them as and the objects and practices they will remember them by. Thus the notes can be considered agents that have the ability to change the living as persons. We will illustrate this point by providing examples of what their authors hoped the notes would accomplish. This could be practical aspects, including instructions that they would not like to be resuscitated, what the funeral should be like, and the distribution of their possessions. Desired outcomes could also include how they would like the bereaved person to react to the suicide and how the deceased person would like to be remembered.

General material and practical aspects

The notes were used to convey messages to the bereaved, including consolations, exhortations and accusations, but also instructions. In this regard, the notes covered a whole range of human emotions and communications. Most straightforward were those notes that informed the person discovering the body – especially if the deceased expected the arrival of the emergency services – of the deceased person's name and the contact details of their next of kin. Other notes instructed those who found them that they did not want to be resuscitated, because they did not want to live. One note urged the police to investigate criminal activities that the deceased person claimed to know about.

Funerals

In eight instances the notes contained instructions about the deceased person's funeral. The most common request was to be cremated, followed in some cases by instructions about what should happen with the ashes. This trend towards cremation is in keeping with the rising popularity of this form of disposal (Hockey *et al.*, 2007). Nonetheless, one deceased person specified that not only did they want to be buried rather than cremated, but that their favourite fluffy toys and a packet of cigarettes and a lighter should find their way into the coffin. The authors of the suicide notes also made requests about the form their funeral should take, such as being 'small', or 'happy – no suits etc' or that the bereaved should give them 'a good send off.' They also specified friends or ministers who should give a reading or say a few a words. Music also featured in these notes. In one instance, the note itself contained a few lines of the song 'Seasons in the Sun', in another the deceased person asked for a particular piece of music to be played at the funeral. 'Time of your Life (Good Riddance)' by the Californian punk band Green Day was requested, as were Bach's Second Piano Concerto and the last record of UK pop group Steps.

Distribution of possessions

The authors of the suicide notes were not only concerned about the form of their disposal, but some also had views about what should happen with their possessions. In one case the deceased person explained that they had set aside money to help with the costs of the funeral. Directives of what should happen after their death also included finding a good home for the deceased persons' pets, with suggestions made as to who would be most suitable or most willing to look after the animals. More commonly, suicide notes offered instructions as to how possessions amongst bereaved family members and friends should be divvied up. In doing this, the deceased person demonstrated consideration of what the recipient might enjoy or would be of use to them.

The items that were distributed in this way were objects that the deceased person considered to be valuable. This could be monetary value, such as houses, cars, or video recorders, stereos and other entertainment electronics, but the value could also be in terms of the enjoyment the recipient might derive from this gift, as in the case of DVDs or CDs, or books or other objects:

> Cherubs in bathroom with dresses [female name] would love them. Bridal chair on landing [son's partner] has always admired it, plus Auntie's silver.
> (Case 38)

Some items could combine several of the above qualities, and in addition also possess sentimental value. This was especially the case for jewellery:

> The brooch/earrings belonged to my mummy – they're not valuable but I always thought it was fun and pretty.
> The plain gold cufflinks were given to me when I was a teenager and belonged to my grandfather (my father's father) who wore them lots!
> (Case 72)

In this case the deceased person used objects to ensure his continuing relationship with his son. Not only did he pass on a memento, but he also provided some explanation for his child that turned him and the child into members of a lineage or kin group that was stretching across several lifetimes. By distributing valuable or meaningful possessions amongst their bereaved family and friends, the deceased person demonstrated consideration over who they considered best suited to receive these gifts. Robert Hertz has argued that death challenges the social order and that funeral rituals are a way to repair the damage that has been caused to society by the loss of one of its members (Hertz, 1960). Under these circumstances, distributing the deceased person's possessions is a way to reintegrate both the deceased person and the bereaved kin into the society, the former as an ancestor, and the latter by taking over the place and roles the deceased person occupied before their death. The crucial difference between Hertz's scenario and the suicide notes that contained instructions for the distribution of possessions was that who receives what was not a collective decision, based on traditional rules, but an individual one – by the deceased person with the recipient in mind. This means that passing on objects had not only the potential to recreate social unity, but also division.

Emotional aspects

The note's intended effect was not restricted to material or pragmatic aspects, but included attempts to influence the emotional state of the bereaved persons. In particular, the majority of the notes tried to make the bereaved feel better about the death, by insisting that their actions had no, or only negligible, impact on the deceased person's decision to take his or her life. There may be a statement that the suicide was unavoidable and no-one's fault (including the deceased). This denial of agency effectively makes the suicide appear to be the choice of no choice. So when an elderly man decided to kill himself, he wrote in the note to his family:

> But my time has come
> I want you to be happy for me.
> I couldn't have wished for a better family you are the BEST!!!
> (Case 6)

Influencing the way the bereaved felt about the death sometimes concerned relationships between members of the bereaved family.

For instance, the woman in Case 38 stressed in her letter to her husband that he had been a wonderful husband even though 'we have grown apart, both ending up hating each other and still caring very much.' The couple had been about to separate, but nonetheless she emphasised in her note to her son that he should not 'think this has anything to do with your father. I have always loved you back both very much. Please be strong for him this is only because of my many health problems and loving you both very much.' In this instance, the letters tried to ameliorate potential conflict between father and son, though her reference to the relationship difficulties she was experiencing with her husband may in fact have reinforced suspicions that it was central to her decision to end her life. More controversially, suicide notes could also be used to create or exacerbate conflict between members of the bereaved family. We have already mentioned the case where the deceased person had asked a former spouse to refrain from exercising her right as his next of kin when it came to his inheritance. Yet even in the case of acrimonious relationships, such as this one, did the deceased person begin his suicide note by urging his former wife not to feel guilty, because 'the situation between us merely hastened things along. I always intended to take my own life one day'.

Hence, the deceased persons tried to influence the emotional states of the living, the way they accounted for or explained the death, and the way that relationships between them developed. However, that the deceased persons' ability to intervene was limited was exemplified by the touching letter a mother left for her son (Case 65). She wished for him to have a happy childhood with his adoptive parents and explained to him that she was suffering from bad depression and was unable to face another day. This did not mean that she did not want him, she emphasised, only that she was ill and could not give him the care he needed. She finished by asking him to remember that he was a wanted child and very much loved. At the same time, she only expected him to receive her letter when he came of legal age, nearly a decade after her death.

Conclusion

This chapter has progressed by honing in on different aspects of suicide notes that allow them to become conduits through which the deceased person can exercise agency. We want to finish off by making a plea for the sociological autopsy as an approach that allows for the incorporation of a wider social and cultural context of suicide and against studying suicide notes in isolation. Our examples of suicides notes largely illustrate how affecting, heart-felt, and magnanimous many of them were. Sanger and McCarthy Veach (2008) have also commented on how positive relationship themes were more prevalent than negative ones and they speculate that the consideration of the finality of the impending suicide allowed the authors to acknowledge the positive relationships in their lives. This may be true, but it is also possible – and our data support this view – that in some cases the overt expression of positive relationships was intricately linked with significant absences. The father who left heirloom jewellery to his son (Case 72) had recently been asked for a divorce by his wife. At that moment he told her that they would discuss the matter in two weeks time. When he was found dead eight days later he was surrounded by photographs of his children, who were also the recipients of his suicide note, together with other mementos. He did not leave a note to his wife, nor any possession, and he had transferred all money from a bank account that he held jointly with his wife into one in the name of his children. Similarly, a woman aged 91 wrote a touching note full of gratitude for the kindness of family and friends:

> I want to find [male name] again, for that is where my happiness is. I think I have had a lovely life here, especially with my grandchildren. I hope that what I now own will be honestly shared among all four. The greatest gift of all. Many thanks to everyone who has given me wonderful support especially in this corner of [*Town*], but I need to be with my man of 64 years. If, when you read this, I should still be alive, please let me go on my journey and please remember [female name], a friend indeed.
> (Case 22)

Yet there was no mention of her daughter with whom she had fallen out, nor did the daughter benefit from any inheritance. Thus the notes were not only about connecting but they also perpetuated old disconnections. Our intention in highlighting this aspect is not to speak ill of the dead, but to act as a reminder that much of the distress surrounding suicide derives from it being fundamentally ambiguous and riven with contradictions. Any research into suicide would do well to work with this quality rather than trying to ignore it or hide behind neat categories.

6
Repertoires of Action

The previous two chapters have both shown how the contents of suicide files are shaped by the broader social context in which the suicide occurs. Our focus in this chapter shifts as we begin to use the contents of the files to explore the lived experiences of suicidal individuals and the circumstances in which suicides take place. Ultimately we hope to be able to say something about causality though, in so doing, we will retain our interest in meaning and motivation. Following the likes of Cavan (1965 [1928]) and Douglas (1967) we take the view that the interpretive or subjective dimension is crucial to explaining suicidal behaviour. What Blumer (1956, 1969) describes as a 'stimulus-response' model of causation is, we argue, of limited value in the study of suicide, not least because of the importance of the interpretive dimension and the complexity of the circumstances in which such action typically occurs. Advocating a more subtle psychosocial approach, we use the idea of 'repertoires of action', to argue that individual suicidal events can best be understood by the changing relationship people have to their perception of their situation, the perception they have of themselves and the perception they have of what people like them – in their situation – might reasonably do. Drawing on fairly detailed accounts taken from the sociological autopsy study our analysis begins to explore the relationship between the individual, the circumstances they perceive themselves to be in and the suicidal act.

According to Douglas (1967) the main problem with established theories of suicide and their reliance on official statistics is the assumption that suicidal actions have a uni-dimensional meaning. This error, he contends, is a function of the basic weakness of the 'statistical-hypothetical' or 'positivistic' approach: namely, the failure to recognise that social meanings are fundamentally problematic. In a similar vein, the analysis presented below draws attention to the complexity and ambiguity of the circumstances in which suicide is typically enacted. Our central argument is that the isolation of one problem or dominant issue that is present in a suicide is rarely, if ever, sufficient to explain the event. Based on the cases we examined it does not appear to be the case that any suicide is caused by one thing in isolation. If this were the case we would expect people who share a feature associated with suicide to all behave in similar ways, but they do not. This is, of course, because similar events or experiences are interpreted differently by different people and because of other features in their lives that they do not share. We argue that it is social actors' relationship to the network of events and issues that they perceive as present in their situation that establishes the range of behaviours that they deem reasonable and appropriate. In some circumstances suicide is one option that can seem a reasonable response to a set of circumstances for a particular person – and this view is subjectively situated. Others may not think suicide is a reasonable response, but, ultimately, it is the individual themselves who determines the appropriateness of a range of behavioural options. This situated and subjectively-oriented range of options is what we refer to as 'repertoires of action'. As will be explained below, this is a term more familiar in the study of new social movements, but we have adapted it to shed light on the behaviour of individuals in distress.

To demonstrate the subjectively situated nature of suicide we have used a case-based approach which provides a detailed examination of a small number of cases.[4] The best known approach to the study of

---

[4]Case studies were selected to reflect distinctive themes across the life-course. The importance of a life-course perspective was confirmed by the statistical analysis of the 100 cases (see Chapter 7), but was also evident from our initial reading of the files in the coroner's office. In particular, we became aware that young people did not in fact dominate the data set as popular understandings of suicide would predict and there were, in fact, very many cases of suicides of people in mid-life. Formal statistical analysis also indicated that there are distinctive associations at different stages of the life-course: for example, young people experiencing problems in childhood and suicide attempts; people in mid-life having problems related to work and family; and older people experiencing ill health and bereavement. The four cases which we highlight in this chapter illustrate these life-course themes, which will then be discussed more thoroughly in Chapter 7.

individual suicides is the psychological autopsy, pioneered in the United States by Schneidman (1969, 1994a) and since applied in numerous countries (see Hawton *et al.*, 1998; Cavanagh *et al.*, 2003). A key criticism of such studies is the tendency to weight consider-ations of cases away from possible social explanations for action towards psychiatric antecedents (Gavin and Rogers, 2006: 135). A reliance on psychiatric explanations for suicidal events might tell us part of a story but it is inevitably partial. A default ascription of suicide to psychological disturbance might, as Gavin and Rogers suggest, 'do no more than provide common sense answers to what may, in reality be very complex events' (p. 139). These authors cite a particular study based on interviews with relatives of people that had recently killed themselves and where the orientation of invest-igation appears to interrogate both social and psychological reasons for suicide. However, on closer examination they conclude that 'the interview schedule devised for the project makes it abundantly clear that the emphasis throughout was to be on mental health topics' (p. 139). Our study aims to respond to the concern expressed by Gavin and Rogers, attempting to examine the circumstances around individual suicidal events without resorting to either deterministic causal categories or pathologies. Repertoires of actions provided a way of doing precisely this. The focus of the chapter is on providing thick description, within the repertoires of action framework, leading to a more fully theorised account of suicide in Chapter 7.

The concept of 'repertoires of action'

For us, a useful way of thinking about the relationship between an individual and their interpretation of the contexts within which they find themselves was to be found in an unlikely place. The concept of repertoires of action has been used in the study of new social movements, where it has been deployed to aid under-standing of why particular organisations behave in the ways that they do – particularly with regards to strategies and tactics for pro-test. Given our very different subject matter, we have not attempted to directly transpose the concept wholesale but have rather adapted it to further our discussion of the relationship between individuals and social contexts – or more simply the situations in which people find themselves.

The term 'repertoires of action', in its crudest sense, refers to the range of activities that characterise a dominant approach taken by a social movement organisation to promoting change (Carmin and Balser, 2002). In explaining how particular tactics or strategies become part of a repertoire of action, Carmin and Balser (2002: 367) explain:

> The choice of a repertoire of action is shaped by structural factors and socio-political conditions. It is also determined by the shared beliefs, attitudes, and understandings of organizational actors. Organizational members do not merely respond to internal and external conditions but rather engage in a sensemaking process that leads to the development of subjective interpretations of reality.

This perspective explicitly engages with an interpretivist epistemology. Members of groups are said to engage in a sense-making process which develops subjective interpretations of reality. As two people in broadly similar circumstances might have very different orientations towards the possibility of suicidal behaviour, so environmental organisations might have similar environmental philosophies but very different action strategies.

The key tenets in formulating repertoires of action – or the strategies of acceptable thoughts and actions – for social movements are, according to Carmin and Balser (2002), four fold: 1) experience; 2) core values and beliefs; 3) environmental philosophy; and 4) political ideology. These four 'cognitive filters', as Carmin and Balser call them, are said to be inter-related, but are presented separately for conceptual clarity.

Repertoires of action and suicide

Taking a theory that was developed for making sense of organisations and applying it to individual behaviour presents obvious challenges. Nonetheless, we would suggest that the usefulness of the concept of repertoires of action for our purposes lies, firstly, in the combination of subjective meaning-making and social structures and, secondly, in the idea that the menu of potential actions available to someone will expand or contract according to their beliefs and social circumstances. The concept provides a useful framework for starting to think about the meaning that suicidal individuals may be attaching to their position in a nexus of circumstances.

In order to understand why suicide becomes a conceivable option to somebody it is necessary to examine the immediate circumstances they were in when they killed themselves, look at the experiences which led to them being in these circumstances and relate these two elements to the values and beliefs the person held which might support suicidal action. It is then possible to examine the repertoires of action that were apparent to the individual at the time of their death. In what follows, we outline our adaptation of Carmen and Balser's theory for individuals in distress.

1. Clusters of circumstances

If we contend that suicides are complex and relational to many aspects of a person's life, it is necessary to examine the multiple circumstances that are present at the time of their suicide. Suicides always seem to contain multiple elements. The extent to which particular elements are more significant than others can be contentious, but it is important to recognise that accessing those factors that are contributory will help enrich any claims made about how the suicidal event came about.

Rather than focusing on a narrow range of factors, we think it might be more useful to consider the nexus of circumstances a person is in. This nexus should be considered dynamic, moreover, and may change in ways that produce different perceptions or outcomes. If the relationship between the suicidal individual and their circumstances is so interwoven, and subjectively constituted, the question of establishing any straightforward uni-causal or stimulus-response model of causality becomes problematic. How can suicides be explained if we do not have knowledge of individuals' changing relationship to a nexus of circumstances? A momentary change to a perception of circumstances might provoke one person to suicide and another to a different course of action (Johnson and Fincham, 2008). To put it another way, our focus is on how an individual's network of circumstances might open doors to suicide, rather than on isolating a limited range of risk factors which are seen to cause suicide via a deterministic stimulus-response relationship.

2. Experience

It is through experiences, and importantly the meanings individuals attach to experiences that they get a sense of strategies that they believe will best serve their purposes in any given situation – in the context of suicide this often includes combinations of things like the amelioration of suffering, the avoidance of shame or guilt, the punishing of others etc. Experience involves the selection of strategies that are known to be effective through previous deployment. However, it also incorporates the idea that some strategies or perceptions individuals have are borne out of the disillusionment with the perceived failure of strategies adopted in previous situations. The utility of experience is in gauging what has worked in the past, how then to manipulate circumstances to a desired end or the realisation that particular strategies have not worked, thus provoking the development of new strategies – perhaps more radical or extreme than before. This may help to explain the pattern of escalation, whereby actual suicide follows a series of previous failed attempts.

3. Values and beliefs

Social actors hold normative views about what should be rather than what is. Reference to the values of the deceased in coroners' case files can be either explicit or implicit. When values shift out of consciousness they are transformed into tacit beliefs and assumptions – individuals construct their reality on the basis of these beliefs and assumptions, and if they appear to be supported by external 'realities' they become deeply engrained. Obviously profound values and beliefs have a bearing on the individual's assessments of the appropriateness of various actions. In terms of analysis, this is the strength of a social scientific approach. An individual's interpretation of particular situations or implicit values or beliefs provides the basis for theorising and connections to social scientific concepts permit a richer examination of suicides than a simple description of surface phenomena.

4. Repertoires of action

Through the exercise of values and beliefs, individuals construct ideas about the ideal relationship between themselves and their social context. Repertoires of action come about through individual's view of the situation they find themselves in (cluster of circumstances), their reflections on the success of previous strategies they have employed (experience) and their views on what matters (values and beliefs). The assessment of reasonable behaviour that arises from these three elements creates a repertoire of action. This is not a deterministic schema and may contain various choices, albeit ones that are constrained by the circumstances in which they are made. Nonetheless, the subjective component remains central because it helps to explain differences in behaviour of people who are in apparently similar situations. For some, suicide becomes a reasonable course of action because of their view of their circumstances, their experiences and because of their values and beliefs. For others it does not.

Case studies

'Daniel' (case 27)

Daniel was an 18-year-old male student who died by hanging. From the police report of sudden death we are told that Daniel had changed his surname to his mother's maiden name. We are also told he had recently separated from his girlfriend and that the night after arguing with her he had hanged himself. The report concludes with the comment that Daniel's parents were estranged and that he is thought to have been depressed 'for some time'.

The coroner's report stated that Daniel had been living with his grandfather, Alan, for well over a year due to domestic problems at his parental home. In another statement it turned out that Daniel's mother, Anne, was also living at Alan's house.

In an interview with Daniel's grandfather, a picture is painted of a popular student and talented athlete. Daniel had a girlfriend, Jody, and they had talked about getting married after their studies. The weekend before Daniel's death, Alan had sent him and Jody to London to see a show for Jody's birthday. The implication from the grandfather was that there was nothing discernibly wrong with Daniel in the months and weeks leading up to his suicide. However, on the Friday before his death there was an incident where Daniel did not turn up to a pre-arranged venue to get a lift with his grandfather. Jody phoned later and was surprised that he was not at home. An hour after the phone call Daniel arrived home obviously distressed and went straight to bed. He refused to talk about where he had been or what he had been doing. This was the last time that Alan saw his grandson alive.

In the grandfather's statement it was also revealed that Daniel had refused to go to work at his part-time job on the Saturday before his death and this was unusual. The day before the discovery of Daniel's body, Alan and Anne went out shopping. When they returned there was a note from Daniel to his mother saying 'sorry I didn't tell you I'm stopping out tonight. Don't be mad, love Daniel'. This was not unusual as Daniel had been known to leave notes telling Alan and Anne of his intentions and he often stayed at Jody's house.

Daniel was not a drinker, did not like parties much and did not indulge in any form of recreational drug taking as far as his family knew. Alan ended his statement by saying that Daniel was very secretive about school and his private life and would not volunteer any information about either. Alan had bought Daniel a car about nine months before his death which Daniel had crashed two months later.

There is also an interview with Jody in the coroner's file. In it she says that Daniel was shy amongst strangers but a 'leader' amongst his circle of friends, and she corroborates the grandfather's observation of Daniel's athletic prowess. A little more than a year before his death, Jody noticed a change in Daniel's mood and said that he became totally dependent on being around her. She believed that this was due to his parent's domestic problems. She then reports that Daniel cut himself off from his friends and wanted her to do the same.

Jody said that she was aware Daniel had been taking anti-depressant medication. He decided to stop taking the medication several months before his death, telling Jody the pills did not do anything and he did not need them. Just two months before his death Daniel claimed to have taken an overdose of paracetamol tablets as he wanted to die. Despite Jody's best efforts, he refused medical aid. He continued to tell her that he wanted to die 'and he was really down at that time'.

In the week before his death Daniel said 'some very hurtful things' to Jody, but he went to her house one evening and apologised for what he had said. He 'broke down' when she showed him the gift she had intended to give him for his birthday. Jody also told him of a surprise holiday that his father had booked for all of them and Daniel appeared pleased that his father was aiming to 'build bridges'. This exchange concluded with Daniel saying that he wanted to be happy and that he would try and get help. Later that day, after an exam, his mood had changed completely and he appeared 'lost and confused'.

It was Jody's birthday party the next day – the day before Daniel's body was discovered – and Daniel said that he 'would rather die' than go to it. He then told Jody he did not want to see her. Later she rang him and he said that he had taken a large overdose of tablets, she should leave him alone and that he wanted to die. She tried ringing back but he would not answer.

That evening Daniel did in fact go to the party but appeared depressed and confused. He was not with Jody and she reports that he was jealous of her friendships with other people. He was not drunk but was asked to leave by Jody's mother after throwing a punch at another male guest. That was the last time Jody saw Daniel.

Cluster of circumstances

The relational and multi-faceted dimensions of suicidal events are important in getting a sense of how suicide comes to be included within an individual's repertoire of action. In Daniel's story there are many factors present at the time of his death that conspire in such a way as to set the context for suicide. The acrimonious break-up of his parents' relationship caused Daniel anguish, to the point where he changed his surname to his mother's name presumably to distance his identity from that of his father. He appears to have become increasingly introspective, placing pressure on an intimate relationship that at the time of his death seems to have been at breaking point. He had been diagnosed as depressed and had then decided that medication was not effective and stopped taking it. At the time of his death he was in the middle of examinations, a time of increased stress and anxiety for students. There are also a couple of other factors that are not prominent in the construction of the coroner's reports but are present nonetheless. For example, a car accident is mentioned, which could be viewed as coincidental to the suicidal outcome, but as it is proximate to the event it may be reasonable to view it as contributory. There is also the claim of at least one previous attempt at suicide. Whilst this is not an exhaustive list, it does at least begin to illustrate the multi-factorial nature of this particular death.

Experience

There seem to be several features that determine Daniel's view of his experiences and the strategies that he employs to manage these experiences. The most striking is an increasing isolation from familial and wider social relationships on the one hand and an intensification of emotional investment in a single intimate relationship on the other. Throughout the narratives in the file, the reported sociability of Daniel is not evident at the end of his life. Whilst his grandfather portrays him as popular and his girlfriend a leader of a circle of friends this does not appear to be the case at the point when he dies. He has perhaps retreated from family on the basis of experiencing those relationships as difficult. Also, whilst we have little information about his peer group, we can perhaps speculate that he did not use his peers as a source of resilience, possibly because he interpreted his experience with friends in a negative light or at least he did not see his relationships with friends as something to sustain him in difficult times.

Another important experience for the purposes of understanding a repertoire of action is Daniel's reaction to his diagnosis of depression. He acknowledged that he was not well when telling his partner that he wanted to get better, but he was not convinced that medication was a solution to his problems. His suicide could be seen as an outcome of the realisation that desired change is not occurring. In terms of strategies employed by Daniel that emanate from experience, his trajectory into suicide is marked by various types of violence. There is an abstracted violence in the car crash and then, at the end of his life, there is a less abstracted relationship to violence – verbal abuse of his partner, a physical assault of a guest at his partner's party and then his own hanging. His willingness to be violent appears to increase.

Values and beliefs

As has been noted, in our treatment of values and beliefs it is important to recognise both the implicit and explicit expression of both. Clearly there is a certain amount of surmising that has to take place when talking about implicit values or beliefs. However, we believe this is where social science can be useful for framing empirical evidence in wider social and theoretical contexts.

In relation to Daniel, we have a sense from the case file that his isolation was largely self-imposed, and that he wanted his girlfriend to cut herself off from her circle of friends too. This isolation may have been a reaction to the emotional distancing that goes on when families disintegrate – emotional isolation in this sense becomes a defensive strategy against what can happen to previously close relationships. However, for Daniel there is perhaps a desire to maintain a relationship with his girlfriend that reflects the 'ideal' or 'pure' intimate relationship (Giddens, 1992), however undesirable this may have seemed to his ex-partner. His confusion comes to a head with the rather chaotic abuse and remorse cycle he gets into in the last few days of his life. His strategies for managing his relationships, by this point, have not worked. The expressions of a desire to die and claims of previous suicide attempts point to a willingness to view suicide as a legitimate course of action, particularly as other interventions (e.g. prescribed medication) did not change the way he felt.

There may also be a complex relationship to masculinity in Daniel's story. There is the issue of his relationship to his father and his desire to distance himself from a key masculine figure in his life by changing his name, though we are also told this relationship had more recently improved. His relationship with his girlfriend appears to have been increasingly predicated on his desire for exclusivity, which could perhaps be understood as gendered controlling behaviour (see also Chapter 7).

Repertoire of action

The idea that problems in childhood resonate in particularly traumatic ways is of course nothing new. Childhood problems are purported to be present in many suicides (particularly abuse in childhood, see Silverman *et al.*, 1996). Daniel had also reported previous suicide attempts. Both of these issues – difficulties in childhood and a history of suicide attempts – are associated with younger suicides in our study, as will be shown in the next chapter. However, suicide comes to be seen as a reasonable response only in the context of the nexus of circumstances surrounding the person at the time of their death, their perception of experiences that they have deemed successful or unsuccessful and their values and beliefs. For Daniel, problems in childhood and previous suicidal intent need to be seen alongside the challenging effects of family breakdown, perhaps a challenge to an ontologically secure sense of masculine identity, the intensification of particular relationships and the subsequent breakdown of these, a determination that he was unwell but that medication could not help, an inability to manage his feelings and a particularly stressful event – an exam – on the day of his death.

These worked together to develop a situation where suicide became a reasonable and realistic option for an 18-year-old student.

'James' – (Case 48)

James was a 49-year-old civil servant who took an overdose. The report of death – a formal document prepared for the coroner by the coroners' officers in advance of an inquest – stated that he had been recently divorced and had two children who were both adult at the time of James's death. It is reported that for the majority of their married life, James and his wife Sarah had been happy and that 'the deceased was a dedicated family man and appeared to dote on his family'.

According to the file both James and Sarah appeared to be 'social drinkers' however a few years before his death it is reported that James began to drink more heavily and became increasingly violent towards Sarah. On one occasion he was arrested. His son had to intervene, which damaged their relationship to the point that the son would not speak to James. Following this, James and Sarah separated and then Sarah started divorce proceedings. Around this time James was arrested for drink-driving. Witness statements tell us that they 'remained friends' after the divorce but James continued to drink and would telephone Sarah several times a week, often asking her to 'go back with him'. She would decline his offers. A few months before James's death, Sarah started a relationship with a man called Mike. During these few months James telephoned Sarah on several occasions threatening to take his own life as he thought he had 'lost everything'. She would speak to him on the telephone or drive to his home to 'talk him round'.

Having got particularly drunk the day before his death, James called his wife and his daughter and threatened to kill himself. They decided to leave him 'as he had used this type of behaviour in the past to seek attention from family members'. On the day of his death Sarah had arranged for James and her new partner to socialise together. When they had not heard from him on the next day they let themselves into the house and found James dead.

There was a note on James's medical history that stated he was taking medication for heart problems, he had high blood pressure and also suffered from depression. The pathology report concluded that James had overdosed on a combination of heart medication and an anti-depressant.

Sarah, James's ex-wife, gave a witness statement to the police immediately after the discovery of the body:

> I would describe James as a great family guy, he was very happy with family life and he loved being a father. Amy [*daughter*] was a 'Daddy's girl'. He doted on both the children. James likes routine and was very house proud. He used to like cooking and ironing. We had a shared marriage for all the domestic chaos. James was a controlling person, looking back, I can see it was subtly done. He used to make decisions in a way that didn't make him seem authoritative. He wasn't nasty, he used to make you believe you made the decision, but he did. I was happy to go along with him, I was happy with our marriage. I would say that James is a hypochondriac. He would be at the Doctors for any little thing. He had a pre-paid prescription and it was cheaper. James was aware of this and we would laugh together about things.

It seems as though the two of them drank quite heavily, but he started to drink before going to work this spiralled into violence towards Sarah. She said in her statement he could be 'like Jekyll and Hyde'. It is also reported by Sarah that he 'smashed up' the family home a few weeks before he died. After James left the family home their daughter tried to maintain contact, but Sarah acknowledged that the separation affected them differently: 'I had got over the split and was carrying on with my life. I had the children, cats, dogs etc., and he in effect had nothing to occupy him'. Sarah described James as having a difficult relationship with his parents. Following the separation, he went to live with his parents for a while, but on one occasion 'beat his father after he had been drinking' so had to leave. He started then to receive alcohol counselling. Sarah reported:

> James said that his drinking could be linked to something that occurred in childhood that he kept buried. James would get angry and wouldn't talk about it.

There is also a witness statement from Amy, the daughter of James and Sarah. The picture she paints is one of both her mother and father drinking far too much and arguing with each other, though she was obviously extremely fond of him. In contrast to the account given by the ex-wife and her partner, Amy says that her father was very unhappy with Sarah having a new relationship and did not like the new partner.

Cluster of circumstances

Whilst it would appear that James had been leading a relatively 'normal' life, it seems to have unravelled at great speed. The circumstances that surrounded the suicide again speak to the multitude of factors that are influential in the resultant death. For James there was a recent divorce and his ex-wife beginning an intimate relationship with another man. Many of the difficulties are attributed in the file to alcohol abuse. He is diagnosed with other health problems, namely depression and high blood pressure. The end of James's life is punctuated by bouts of violence, towards his wife and his father. The violence appears to have led to an estrangement from his son, while his daughter remained in contact with him. He is also arrested for drink driving. For a man that had been a happy, doting family man just a few years before, the network of circumstances that he found himself in would result in him developing an orientation to ever more extreme thoughts and rationales for 'appropriate' behaviours.

Experience

The passage of James's life appears to follow what many might consider a 'normal' trajectory until the years immediately preceding his death. He is said to have been a happily married man (although the subtly controlling behaviour is noted) and is said to have doted on his family. The centrality of his family to his happiness is repeated several times throughout the accounts of his life from various sources. However, as the family slips away, James continues to drink with increasingly destructive consequences. What is described as 'social drinking' by James and his wife appears to take on a degenerative role in their relationship and violence then becomes a prominent feature of their lives with each other, possibly also being linked to his controlling behaviour.

With the deterioration of the relationship, separation and divorce were initiated by Sarah. It may have been that James could not contain his frustration with the derailing of the sense that he had of the ideal of 'the family' drifting away. To exacerbate this, the behaviour of James clearly affected their son who eventually wanted nothing to do with his father. Their daughter however attempted to maintain contact – perhaps acting as a conduit between the life James used to have and the life he then found himself with. The final couple of years of James's life are punctuated by dramatic problems – notably his arrest for drink driving and a violent assault on his own father. There are glimpses of a deeper malaise buried in James's past that are alluded to by his ex-wife – in particular an incident that James was unwilling to talk about despite attributing his destructive behaviour to his inability to come to terms with whatever it was. His disillusionment with the failure of his attempts at retrieving his previous life led to the development of increasing aggression and violence.

On the day before his death James issued a specific threat to take his own life but unlike other occasions both his ex-wife and daughter chose not to respond because they said 'he had used this type of behaviour in the past to seek attention from family members'. In a sense, this case illustrates the problems with the popular myth that people who are going to kill themselves will just go and do it (rather than talking about it). James did talk about killing himself on several occasions, but this time, possibly as a response to not getting the desired attention from his wife or daughter, he took decisive action.

Values and beliefs

For James, the idea of family appears to be important, as do the ideas of order and control. The ideal of a strong family is confounded by the reality of deterioration in his marriage and his relationship with his son. Different relationships appear to become increasingly problematic or complicated once the certainties in James's life are undermined. This process includes separation from a wife that he professed to want to reconcile with, estrangement from his son after he intervened in a violent assault against his mother, continued contact – and sympathy – from his daughter and a relationship with his own parents that resulted in violence apparently exacerbated by alcohol. There is also the introduction of another man in the life of his ex-wife. There is a reorientation of James's strategies towards more extreme behaviour as his values and beliefs are undermined and new ones emerge, perhaps with emotional difficulties in relation to a troubling experience from the past and loss of control – graphically represented by drinking and the consequences associated – being a prominent feature of the last few months of his life.

If alcohol, violence and depression might be identified as obvious explicit explanatory features of James's death there is another aspect which requires a social scientific interpretation. It is difficult to ignore the gendered nature of James's difficulties in accepting particular roles within the network of circumstances that emerge towards the end of his life. James seems to have been subtly controlling (his wife's term) within the family, perhaps in the service of maintaining a particular role as husband and father. Throughout the story of James each of the key tenets of his role as a family man are undermined, culminating in jealousy of his wife's new relationship. Running concurrent with this challenge to his sense of masculinity is his implicit inability to accept responsibility for the situation in which he found himself. It is interesting to note the symbolic gesture of a man described as 'houseproud' smashing up the house in the weeks before his death – this seems to represent the acting out of the destruction of his idea of 'home' as his concept of family dissolves around him.

Repertoire of action

For James it appears as though the nature of his social location in the last few years of his life involved a persistent and, perhaps to him, inexorable undermining of what Goffman (1959) would describe as a sense of a competent social identity. This related to the increasing violence and chaos that James found himself in, this for a man that is described by his wife as liking control and who placed a high value on family. The sense of loss, displacement and dislocation speaks to the social and relational as much as the psychological. The relationship to alcohol, gender, family, age, the law and a troubling childhood history all are present in the circumstances that create a situation for James to consider killing himself. It is not possible to ascertain, or talk simplistically about a mechanical relationship between one or two of these circumstances, or to suggest that the suicide is simply the result of a disturbed state of mind. The various elements work together to allow for particular repertoires of action to emerge. Eventually this repertoire included suicidal behaviour. This was initially only the threat of suicide, but in fact serious suicidal intent seems to have lain behind the threats which were interpreted as manipulative. Finally, perhaps in response to his plea for attention being ignored, he took an overdose which killed him.

'Carol' (Case 54)

Carol was a 43-year-old woman who overdosed at home. The report of death tells us she was divorced and her GP described her as drinking and being depressed. Under 'medical history', the report of death simply notes that she had being diagnosed with depression and had previously self-harmed. The forensic report details Carol's prescription regimes which included a herbal remedy, a tricyclic anti-depressant, a benzodiazepine and a compound analgesic which contained an opiate. Carol's partner, Tony, explained the context of their relationship in his witness statement. They had known each other for about 20 years but had lost touch in that time and then regained contact. They started a relationship three years before Carol's death.

Tony described Carol as 'a happy person' who 'had a few health problems', including depression and 'problems with her back and left breast'. Her back problems resulted in broken sleep and she would often sleep in the afternoons. She was also receiving Hormone Replacement Treatment (HRT) because of 'mood swings'. Tony reported that Carol 'would worry about friends and relatives and money problems quite a lot'. She had worked as a barmaid and waitress in the past, but for the last three years had been on benefits and unable to work because of her back problems. It seems Carol had not seen her children (Emma, Lisa and John) for some time 'after problems when she got divorced', but had re-established contact with them in the last three years.

In Tony's witness statement, there then followed a poignant description of the last time they were to see each other:

> I went into the flat and I saw Carol on her knees in the kitchen. She was emptying the freezer. She had told me the day before that she had no electricity in the flat and needed to remove the food. She had been crying. She was upset. I looked at her face and could see tears in her eyes. She then said to me 'I won't be needing this, if you don't take it I'm going to throw it in the bin'. I replied 'don't be silly', she then repeated her previous comment. I then said 'if you are going to be like that, then I'm going home'. 'I then picked up 3 carrier bags full of food and left the flat. This was the last time that I saw Carol alive.'

In this particular case there were a collection of suicide notes. The notes are opportunities for the person that has died to first give

some sort of account of their perception of their position in relation to the circumstances in which they find themselves, but also
to attempt to control future references to their lives and deaths
(see Chapter 5). In this particular case there are four notes, one
to Carol's partner, one to her children and two very short notes
to the emergency services that might find her.

Suicide note to partner
Hi [*nickname*]
   As I am writing this letter I mean I have not long left as
I shall be writing two more letters one to Emma and one to
John.

When you walk out on Saturday again I knew what I had to
do, I have never loved anyone more than I have loved you
and as I don't or could love anyone else it is time to go. I know
you did not like me going to bed in the afternoon but that was
the only time when I got to have any decent sleep. Well it is
1.30pm you walked in ten minutes ago and took your clothes
and I emptied the freezer for you so the food would not go to
waste I told you I would not be here for long and I meant it
I shall have a bath now and go to sleep and never wake up
again Please look after Kitty [*cat*] for me – remember I always
loved you.
   Carol
PROVED YOU WRONG THIS TIME

Suicide note to daughter and son
Emma and John
   I am so sorry for what I have done but Tony meant so much to
me that I can't live without him while I am writing this I am
taking all my tablets. I am so glad I got to see you get married I
was so proud of you and I am so proud of the way you are bringing Nathan [*grandson*] up. Will you tell John for me and tell him I
am so sorry I did not get to know him as well as I wanted to but I
really did love him even though I did not tell him I did. You see
Emma even though I got you and John and Lisa it is not enough
for me I needed Tony as well and if I can't have him then I don't
want to live I am going to finish now as I want to bath before the

tablets take effect I really am sorry don't blame the medics because I have left a letter saying they are not to do anything other than let me die.

All my love

Mum

xxx

xx

x

Carol left two notes for the emergency services, one stating the dosage of medication she had taken and another saying 'MEDICS DO NOT ATTEMPT TO REVIVE ME I DO NOT WISH TO LIVE'.

Cluster of circumstances

For Carol at the time of her death there were several key factors present that previous studies have found to be often associated with suicide. She was diagnosed with depression and was known to self-harm. In fact these are the two issues highlighted as relevant medical history in the report of death. As with the other cases discussed in this chapter, it is our contention that these 'risk factors' in isolation or even in combination are not enough to explain why a person would kill themselves. Carol suffered from poor physical health and broken sleep. Her health had, it seems, impacted on her capacity to work, compounding concerns she had about money. She had experienced a prolonged separation from her three children, and whilst we are told that there had been a recent reconciliation, this might suggest Carol had to reorient her feelings about the past, as well as the present. There is also the suggestion of difficulties in her relationship with her partner. On the day of her death they had had an argument. Her suicide notes implicate the loss of her partner in her decision to take her life, although it is fairly clear she was already very distressed when he arrived at the house, rather than her distress being initiated by his walking out on her.

Experience

Carol's experience seems to be dominated by the relationship between her ill health – both physical and mental – material concerns (employment, money) and her sense of selfhood in relation to others, in particular her partner and children. Her life is marked by failure in normative expectations – particularly in relationships. She had been divorced, estranged from her children and involved in a turbulent relationship with somebody that she appears to have thought was leaving her. There is a certain sense of hopelessness in the ways in which Carol has dealt with the problems in her life. Her physical ill health, coupled with depression, has resulted in prolonged periods of the day in bed. She was receiving HRT to control what are described as 'mood swings', as well as taking anti-depressants. Her experience of medical treatment and her own ways of coping with ill health do not seem to have led to a positive outlook. Whilst there is not much information indicating how Carol reacted to specific experiences, there are clues in the ways in which she writes about the past in her suicide notes. She acknowledges that she had not managed to convey her feelings to the children with whom she had been relatively recently reconciled and she writes of an overwhelming sense of loss at the prospect of not being with Tony.

Values and beliefs

Carol's values and beliefs are not explicit, but there are indications that her situation fell a long way short of her expectations of a reasonable life. The estrangement from her children, and then the sense that the reconciliation was not enough to keep her alive, might suggest that her depth of attachment was not as great as she might have wanted. In particular she regrets not having a closer relationship with her son John. We are also told that she no longer worked and that she was consistently worried about money. Whilst we do not know much about Carol's personal values and beliefs, we could speculate that perhaps dominant social values, such as the importance of respectability and family ties are challenged by a sense of failure: as a mother, through prolonged estrangement from her children; failure as a wife through divorce; failure as a worker, because of incapacity claims for three years; and, finally, failure as a partner in her current relationship with Tony.

Repertoire of action

We are told that Carol's repertoire of action already involved a willingness to self-harm, although we do not have any evidence about the timing or circumstances of this previous self-harm or how exactly self-harm became one of the options available to her in response to particular events or experiences. We do know something of the multiple problems she faced, as explained above and outlined in her suicide notes. We also know that she 'proved [Tony] wrong' in taking her life. In terms of a repertoire of action, this last statement suggests that her orientation to her circumstances had changed sufficiently for her to carry out something that had been perceived as a hollow threat before.

Throughout the coroner's file on Carol's death there are references to depression being the key feature of the case. Depression might perhaps be the feature highlighted in a psychological autopsy study of the case, since mental illness is the most frequently occurring risk factor identified in these kinds of studies (Cavanagh *et al.*, 2003). However, we would see the multiplicity of difficult social circumstances and psychological responses to these as providing a fuller picture of the suicide than simply an identification of mental illness. Suicidal behaviour does not, of course, occur in all people with multiple health and personal problems; nor does it occur in all people with depression. An inter-disciplinary perspective is required that considers in the round the various different influences on suicidal individuals. Unfortunately, the complexity of social circumstances is often not prioritised, either in research on suicide or in professional processing of deaths by suicide.

'Malcolm' (Case 53)

Malcolm was a 67-year-old man who suffered from Parkinson's disease and depression and who killed himself with an overdose shortly before Christmas. The police reported that he had worked as a self-employed craftsman, but his health had prevented him from working for a number of years prior to his death. His wife had killed herself four years before his death and he had been seen by his GP about bereavement issues. He had recently complained of suffering from vertigo and was on a variety of medication.

Malcolm had a complex medical history since his diagnosis with Parkinson's 13 years earlier. As well as having vertigo he had visited his GP a fortnight before his death complaining of amnesia. According to the consultant pathologist's report at the time of his death he was prescribed two kinds of medication for the Parkinson's, as well as a benzodiazepine, an analgesic and an anti-inflammatory drug. This prescription regime was corroborated by the post mortem toxicology report, but it was in fact a tricyclic anti-depressant that killed him, being 'found in the blood at a concentration consistent with a fatal overdose'.

Malcolm had taken an overdose in the months following his wife's suicide and as a result was prescribed an SSRI anti-depressant. However the GP described Malcolm as 'incompliant'. Later that year, although he was said to be 'suffering from a bereavement reaction', Malcolm's condition appeared to improve dramatically. According to the GP this was 'helped by the implantation of a deep brain stimulator for his Parkinson's Disease [*a number of months since the bereavement*] which had a huge effect on his disease state'.

Some months before his death Malcolm visited the GP complaining of depression and was given a different type of SSRI anti-depressant, as suggested by a Parkinson's specialist. Three months later he returned. The GP reports that Malcolm found the medication 'ineffective and was troubled by its side effects'. Since on that day the GP thought he did not seem depressed, it was agreed that he should 'leave off treatment'. In the month before his death Malcolm was prescribed a benzodiazepine (Temazepam) after complaining of sleep problems.

Another key document in the file is a statement from Malcolm's brother. He had let himself into Malcolm's house with a spare key and discovered the body. In addition to the information noted above, he reported that Malcolm had repeatedly apologised to people about his speech, affected as this was by the Parkinson's disease. He said of Malcolm's wife's suicide that she had been depressed for a long time following her mother's death and that the death of his wife had 'affected Malcolm massively and he perhaps never got over it'. The brother's statement also mentions another person of some significance:

Malcolm had an ex-wife from years ago who resides in the USA. They have been in contact however. He has stated to me that he was upset because she was messing him about. For example she forgot to phone Malcolm on his birthday.

The brother also noted that Malcolm would regularly say he was not happy with his life, saying 'I'm in pain – all I can do is lie in bed'. It also appeared to his brother that Malcolm had been getting his affairs in order for a period of time before his death, implying that he had been planning it for a while:

> Malcolm would state that his head seemed to be getting worse. He felt very dizzy. I am aware that Malcolm changed his will approximately 3 weeks ago. This was because his first wife's details were on it and he decided he didn't want her to receive as much. I am also aware that Malcolm seemed to be preparing for his funeral by saving for various things. I do believe Malcolm's headaches were getting worse and this was affecting his life.

Malcolm left a suicide note which read 'Please I do <u>not</u> want to be kept alive. Too much <u>pain</u>'.

Cluster of circumstances

The dominant features in the coroner's file on Malcolm's suicide are his suffering with Parkinson's and the suicide of his wife four years earlier. It is reasonable to assume that these factors were primary motivators to a suicidal end. However, there are other elements to the story that are worth noting. It is not simply a case of Malcolm reacting to his wife's death by killing himself. There is a period of time between the suicides and in this time we get a sense of the fluctuation of optimism and pessimism that marked Malcolm's life immediately prior to his death. He killed himself just before Christmas. This is a period often associated with heightened distress for people recently bereaved, given its symbolic importance as a time of celebration and family bonding. He was not only suffering from Parkinson's, but was also being treated for amnesia and vertigo. Malcolm had also recently re-established contact with an ex-wife. This relationship was important enough to him that he became upset with her for not remembering his birthday.

Experience

The death of Malcolm's wife appears to have been a key motivator in his reaction to the depth of loss he experienced. His wife had suffered depression after the death of her own mother and Malcolm's suicide looks very similar to that of his wife – namely a suicide that has a strong theme of 'bereavement reaction' and where the method of suicide was an overdose of pills. In terms of an orientation to suicide as a legitimate or reasonable action, Malcolm had a close model in the behaviour of his wife in circumstances that are similar to his own. There is also the issue of Malcolm's Parkinson's disease. For Malcolm, the possibility of recuperation, that appeared to be possible with the deep brain stimulator, was relatively short-lived and he then seemed to be dogged by attendant health issues and perhaps developed a certain fatalism about his health. The frustrated possibility of some kind of relationship with his ex-wife also offers an insight into an increasing sense of disappointment with the circumstances Malcolm found himself in. His brother suggests that Malcolm was upset because his ex-wife was 'messing him about' and had forgotten his birthday. In some senses this reaction validates the disillusionment that accompanied Malcolm to his death. The note left by Malcolm suggests that the pain he was experiencing forced him to suicide, but he was not specific about this pain. It could be that alongside physical pain, the emotional anguish he was experiencing following the loss of his wife and then the more recent disappointment with his ex-wife was another type of pain that provoked suicide. This does not appear to have been a spontaneous act, as his brother suggested that Malcolm had been getting his affairs in order prior to his death. In terms of experience this suggests an attempt to have some control of events after death.

Values and beliefs

There is little explicit evidence about Malcolm's values and beliefs, but there is some relevant information about what might be implicit beliefs. His reaction to the prescription of a second type of SSRI antidepressant may point to a certain acceptance of his depression as being immutable or untreatable. He seemed to believe that nothing could help him manage his physical decline – 'I'm in pain. All I can do is stay in bed'. It is as though Malcolm, once he had become convinced of an inevitable unhappy decline, then started to develop conditions (e.g. amnesia) that could reaffirm this belief and perhaps make suicide a more attractive option than staying alive. Whilst we know very little about the relationship with the ex-wife there is enough to suggest that this was something that was exacerbating Malcolm's sense of isolation or anger with his situation. The changing of his will and subsequent suicide suggest a deliberate set of steps being taken to manage the conditions where suicide can occur in the manner desired by Malcolm. This is not to suggest that his physical deterioration is not a key factor in his death but to note that this is not all that is being used by Malcolm as a resource for him to come a conclusion that suicide was a viable option.

Repertoire of action

As has been mentioned, Malcolm had a model for reacting to bereavement provided by his wife's suicide. In a sense, his wife's death, in the context of depression following bereavement, put suicide on the agenda as a potential response to grief and loss. The ongoing situation with Malcolm's physical and mental health, and particularly the apparent belief – his interpretation from his experience – that conditions would not improve, seems to make the option of suicide open to Malcolm. Two obvious factors that feature in this death are bereavement and physical health problems which, as we note in Chapter 7, seem to be features of suicide in older people in our sample. But the issues of mental ill health and connectedness in other social relationships are also important when a fuller story is told.

Conclusion

So what should we make of the analysis presented in this chapter? The first point to emphasise is that social relationships and the affective dimension feature prominently in the circumstances surrounding suicide. The types of relationship that are implicated are many and various, however, reflecting the inevitably subjective nature of this aspect of inter-personal life. Getting a sense of how relationships are viewed or experienced by people is an important exercise for suicidology and using the idea of repertoires of action allows us to acknowledge the importance of some relationships over others, but also acknowledge that relationships are fluid. Secondly, researchers can never be absolutely certain about all of the elements that have contributed to a person killing themselves. There will always be an element of speculation about aetiology; a fact that is often overlooked in suicidology. The final point to emphasise is that there are no simple, clean, linear explanations that can characterise the decisions of a suicidal individual operating in a network of circumstances. The idea of repertoires of action provides an effective way of describing the range of reasonable options available to individuals at a given point in time. These are mutable and some options may come and go. The model presented here is able to account for this mutability, the differences between people in similar situations and ultimately enables us to capture the relational aspects of suicide more fully.

This chapter acts as something of a bridge between the essentially constructionist readings presented in the previous chapters and the more objectivist reading that is to come. We have begun to use the contents of the coroner's files to explore the lived experiences of suicidal individuals and the circumstances in which suicides take place, but we have done so in a way that emphasises the centrality of meaning and motivation. The four case studies we have featured in this chapter are illustrative of some distinctive characteristics of suicides at different stages of the life-course and prepare the way for what is to follow. In the next chapter we present the results of our quantitative analysis and aim to show how suicide and its associated meanings are structured by broader social relations, paying particular attention to the role of social bonds across the life-course, to the significance of intimate relationships and to gendered patterns of work and family life.

7
When Things Fall Apart – Suicide and the Life-Course

In this final empirical chapter we offer a more objectivist reading than has been provided so far. Detailed quantitative analysis of the 100 cases included in our sociological autopsy is presented alongside a more general assessment of the demography of suicide in England and Wales. What we say here should be read in light of what we have already said in earlier chapters, not least because this should guard against the dangers of reifying the relationships that are described below. The meaning of quantitative analysis cannot simply be read off the relationships that are identified but requires a 'plausible narrative' that links variables together as sequences of comprehensible human action (Reiner, 2007). In seeking to provide such a narrative, we have drawn on the results of our qualitative work, including that presented below, as well as recent developments in life-course criminology and longer standing psychoanalytic perspectives. We begin by describing two murder-suicide cases, which illustrate the way in which we have sought to move from statistical relationships to sequences of comprehensible human action. Neither formed part of our dataset and each was identified after we had developed our analysis, providing some kind of external validity. Both cases attracted considerable media attention, presumably because the murders meant they stood out from the much larger number of suicides that occur each year.

Over a period of several weeks during the summer of 2010 a series of UK press reports charted the violent disintegration of Raoul Moat (see, for example, *The Guardian*, July 6 2010 and July 20 2010; *The Telegraph*, July 9 2010 and July 11 2010; *The Independent*, July 18

2010). According to reports, 37-year-old Moat critically injured his ex-girl friend, killed her lover and shot a policeman shortly after his release from an 18 week prison sentence on charges of assault on a family member. All firearms officers in Northumbria Police service were deployed onto the case, augmented by officers drafted in from other forces, making it one of the 'biggest operations' in the force's history. Amid rumours that he had taken hostages and was threatening to kill members of the public, Moat was eventually tracked down and cornered in an area near Rothbury, where he had holidayed as a child. After a six hour stand-off with armed police, it was reported that Moat had shot and killed himself, though it was subsequently suggested he had done so involuntarily having been shot by police using a tazer whilst holding a shotgun to his head. At 6 foot 3 inches tall, a 'steroid-addicted-body-builder' and a former club doorman, Moat was routinely portrayed as a violent man motivated by jealousy, hatred of the police and anger. According to early reports an entry on his Facebook page read: 'Just got out of jail, I've lost everything, my business, my property and to top it all off my lass of six years has gone off with the copper that sent me down. I'm not 21 and I can't rebuild my life. Watch and see what happens' (*The Guardian*, July 6 2010). In an interview after Raoul Moat's death his estranged older brother was quoted as saying he had come from a 'fairly dysfunctional background with very little maternal affection' and suffered a string of failed relationships in a desperate attempt to form a stable family: 'He was just sitting there in the open, in no cover, crying about the fact he had no family and no dad and that nobody loved him. That was not true' (*The Independent*, July 12 2010).

Two years earlier, the deaths of Brian Philcox and his children revealed a similar mixture of anger, loss and lethal violence. On June 15 2008, 53-year-old Philcox collected his children, Amy aged seven and Owen aged three, from his estranged wife as part of their normal access arrangements and took them to a tourist railway in Llangollen, North Wales. As reported in several national newspapers he then telephoned his wife, telling her he had left a 'present' in the house, sparking a full-scale bomb alert, with bomb disposal officers evacuating the family home and neighbouring houses (*Daily Express*, June 17 2008; *The Sun*, June 17 2008; *Daily Mirror*, June 17, 2008). Philcox is then said to have driven to a remote hillside lane in Snowdonia where he piped exhaust fumes into the car, killing himself and his children. In their attempts to make sense of these events, reporters described Philcox as a 'karate expert'; a man who was prone to violence and who was said to have been accused by his estranged wife of attacking her 19-year-old son from a previous relationship. At the same time, we were told that Brian had lost his first wife to cancer and had raised 'thousands of pounds' for charity; that he was 'a lovely, decent man who would not hurt a fly'; that he had been 'forced' into a divorce he did not want and whose attempts to negotiate the court system in order to gain access to his children had left him 'frustrated at every turn' and 'completely broken'. A neighbour was quoted as having overheard Philcox saying: 'I have lost my wife. I have lost my kids. I am going to lose my house. They can all f*** off. I would rather burn the house than give it to that bitch'.

Although murder-suicides are extremely rare the circumstances surrounding the deaths of Raoul Moat, Brian Philcox and their various victims have something important to tell us about suicide more generally. Suicides are concentrated among men in mid-life – a pattern that we argue is linked to the particular challenges that this stage of the life-course presents when things go wrong and life seems to be falling apart. We begin by laying the conceptual foundations of our argument, drawing on life-course criminology, attachment theory and psychoanalysis, before going on to present the empirical evidence. Official statistics covering England and Wales are used to show that people in mid-life account for a disproportionately large number of suicides and are, along with older people, most at risk of killing themselves. We then begin the detailed analysis of 100 cases by demonstrating how patterns of suicide can be seen to map on to conventional features of a socially structured life-course, with young people in crisis, mid-life gendered patterns of work and family and older people in decline. Particular attention is given to the role of family breakdown, which features strongly in mid-life. By highlighting the particular significance of mid-life, we challenge the conventional wisdom that young people, particularly young men, are most at risk of suicide.

What we say in this chapter involves an inevitable degree of speculation given the limitations of the data, but the general thrust of the argument emerged out of the empirical analysis. Ours was an exploratory look at patterns and we did not approach the field with any particular set of ideas we wanted to test. Although statistical techniques were used, they were applied in a manner that is consistent with what are often held to be the defining characteristics of a qualitative approach: that is, the emphasis was explicitly on generating, rather than testing, hypotheses. We turned to life-course criminology, attachment theory and psychoanalysis only when the empirical analysis was complete and did so on the grounds that they seemed to make sense of our findings.

Social bonds and the life-course

The importance of social integration to suicide rates was established by Durkheim (2002 [1897]) and continues to attract considerable interest (see, for example, Maimon and Kuhl, 2008). Without distinguishing clearly between social integration, social ties and social networks (Berkman, Glass, Brissette and Seeman, 2000) – and we could perhaps add social capital and social bonds – much previous work has highlighted the importance of social relationships and involvement in social institutions to understanding suicide. What has not been fully appreciated in such work, however, is the way social relationships and involvement in social institutions vary across the life-course. Where a life-course perspective has been taken or implied, moreover, the focus has been on young people and the elderly, with little if any specific consideration of those in the intervening stages (see, for example, Hawton and van Heeringen, 2000). This is a troubling omission for several reasons, not least because, as we will see below, it does not sit well with the evidence, which points to a particular concentration of suicides among those in mid-life.

To structure our thinking about the life-course, we have drawn on Laub and Sampson's (2003) age-graded theory of informal social control. Such a selection may initially seem odd, since Laub and Sampson were concerned with crime, not suicide, and aimed to explain why offending behaviour varies across the life-course. Some adaptation is certainly required and, in drawing on this work, we do not mean to imply that suicide should be treated as a criminal offence: our purpose is more analytical than normative and we have come to the view that criminology offers a useful template for thinking about suicide. Suicide can, of course, be thought of as a form of extreme violence to the self and there may be similarities in the aetiology of suicide and certain forms of crime. Suicide, like some criminal acts, may, for example, be symptomatic of high levels of impulsivity and low levels of internal and external control. But more importantly, from our point of view, criminology offers a means of making sense of the 'senseless' and of turning the 'pathological' into the social, doing so, in large part, by attending to the meanings and motivations of the social actors involved. One of the particular strengths of Laub and Sampson's approach is that it takes account of meaning, whilst allowing for the interplay of structure and agency. Echoing Giddens' (1984) theory of structuration, it is argued that 'agential processes' are reciprocally linked to situations and larger structures: that is, situations and structures are said to be partly determined by the choices individuals make, yet simultaneously constrain, modify and limit the choices that are available to them. This interplay between structure and agency is summarised as 'situated choice'.

At the heart of Laub and Sampson's analysis lies the claim that persistence in, and desistance from, crime can be meaningfully understood within the same theoretical framework. Persistence, they note, is explained by a lack of social controls, few structured routine activities and purposeful human agency, while desistance is attributed to a confluence of social controls, structured routine activities and purposeful human agency. What is, perhaps, most significant from our perspective is the emphasis on the role of social ties across all stages of the life-course and on the way that social ties interact with age and life experience. Young people tend to be less socially embedded during adolescence than at any other time in the life-course because the bonds that tie children to family and school have weakened and are yet to be replaced by a new set of adult roles and responsibilities. With the move into adulthood new bonds are created, which are said to provide 'turning points' or changes in situational and structural life circumstances. A good marriage and/or a stable job are specifically identified as having the potential to reshape life-course trajectories by reordering short-term situational inducements to crime and redirecting long-term commitments to conformity. Laub and Sampson's respondents who had desisted from crime were found to be embedded in structured routines and were socially bonded to jobs, wives, children, and significant others, which enabled them to draw on resources and social support from their relationships. Those who persisted, on the other hand, were characterised as 'social nomads' who were seemingly devoid of 'connective structures' at each phase of the life-course, especially those involving relationships that could provide informal social control and social support. Residential, marital and job instability were commonly experienced by respondents who continued to offend, prompting the suggestion that: 'Surely part of this chaos reflects an inability to forge close attachments or make any connection to anybody or anything' (Laub and Sampson, 2003: 194).

Attachment theory and psychoanalysis

Whilst providing a useful template for thinking about suicide, Laub and Sampson's analysis does not directly address psychological dimensions of the social bond and we must look elsewhere for this. Laub and Sampson draw heavily on control theory and Hirschi's (1969) classic formulation, which holds that the social bond is comprised of four elements – attachment, commitment, involvement and belief. Of these, attachment and commitment are most salient to our analysis. Personal attachments to others, Hirschi argues, contain the essence of the conscience or superego and, as well as underpinning the internalisation of norms, refer to the emotional connection that individuals feel towards others, including sensitivity to their opinions, feelings and expectations. Commitment, on the other, hand is considered to be the counterpart of the ego or 'common sense' and refers to the accumulated investment that people have in relationships, activities and objects. Hirschi's formulation owes something to Bowlby, who, along with Ainsworth, has done more than anybody to illuminate the role of attachment.

As colleagues and co-authors of attachment theory, Bowlby and Ainsworth spawned 'one of the broadest, most profound, and most creative lines of research in 20th century (and now 21st century) psychology', providing 'the most visible and empirically grounded conceptual framework' in the fields of social and emotional development (Cassidy and Shaver, 2008: xi). Drawing on psychoanalysis and object relations theory, they developed a 'lifespan developmental theory' (Crowell *et al.*, 2008: 599) based on the making and breaking of affective relations. As noted by Bowlby (1982 [1969]: 208), human attachments play a 'vital role...from the cradle to the grave'. The central tenet of attachment is that the young child needs to develop a secure relationship with at least one primary caregiver for social and emotional development to occur 'normally'. Affectional bonds with the caregiver are based on the child's need for safety, security and protection, so that the infant becomes attached to adults who are sensitive and responsive to them. Bowlby (1973) coined the term 'working models' to explain the cognitive aspects of the process, whereby the infant builds working models of the world, particularly about attachment figures (i.e. who they are, their expected response) and themselves (i.e. perceptions of how acceptable or unacceptable one is to the attachment figure). If the attachment figure recognises the child's need for comfort and protection while respecting the child's need to independently explore the environment, the child will likely develop a working model of self as valued and self-reliant. If the caregiver frequently fails to meet the child's need for comfort and exploration, the child will likely develop a working model of self as unworthy or incompetent. Ainsworth (1967; see also Ainsworth *et al.*, 1978) introduced the concept of the 'secure base' to describe the way in which the child can confidently explore the environment with the active support of a caregiver, safe in the knowledge that this attachment figure is available if any need or question should arise. She also identified different attachment patterns in infants, arguing that secure attachment develops where the primary caregiver is responsive and provides a secure base, but that insecure attachments, which she labelled avoidant and anxious, develop in response to unresponsive, neglectful and/or inconsistent care.

Although attachment theory was initially developed with reference to the infant-caregiver relationship, childhood experiences were thought to have long-term consequences and this has been confirmed by subsequent research (Rutter, 2006; Magai, 2008; Thompson, 2008). Bowlby (1973) maintained that the internal working models developed during infancy and childhood are generalised to other people in the adult's social network and that attachment styles are relatively enduring, though he also recognised that these models might change if relational experiences are inconsistent with expectations. For Ainsworth such continuity means that the secure base is critical to adult-to-adult relationships, as well as to infant-or-child-to-adult relationships, facilitating functioning and competence in other realms of life: there is, she notes (1991: 38):

> ...a seeking to obtain an experience of security and comfort in the relationship with the partner. If and when such security and comfort are available, the individual is able to move off from the secure base provided by the partner, with the confidence to engage in other activities.

The central paradox here is that one can only be securely separate if one feels attached in the first place (Holmes, 2001). As well as providing a secure base, spouses and romantic partners, in their role as trusted attachment figures, offer a safe haven to which the attached person can retreat in times of need.

Adult attachment styles have been formally assessed by Bartholomew (1990), among others, who identified two underlying dimensions, which she conceptualises as 'model of self' (positive v negative) and 'model of others' (positive v negative). Based on these dimensions, four theoretical prototypes of attachment style are identified, namely secure, preoccupied, dismissing and fearful. Research evidence has confirmed that secure attachment is linked to a range of positive outcomes in adulthood, including greater satisfaction in relationships and longer relationships characterised by trust, commitment and interdependence (Fraley *et al.*, 2005). Insecure attachment styles among adults and young people have, by contrast, been found to be particularly prevalent among high risk groups (clinical populations and children who have been maltreated or institutionalised) though they are also sufficiently common in 'normal' or low risk groups that they cannot be considered a disorder in their own right (Hesse, 2008; Crowell *et al.*, 2008; Rutter, 2008). Nonetheless, insecure attachment styles have been linked to a range of psychosocial difficulties among adults, including chronic anxiety about rejection and abandonment in close relationships; intimacy anger, jealousy and mood instability; dissociative symptoms and anxiety disorders; domestic violence and other offending-behaviour (Gilchrist *et al.*, 2003; Dozier *et al.*, 2008; Fraley *et al.*, 2005). The 'new' crime of stalking has also been described as a pathology of attachment and attributed to a combination of distal and proximal factors: early attachment disruption, such as the loss or disruption of a primary caregiver relationship, has been identified as a predisposing factor, while recent adult loss, such as the breakup of an intimate relationship or marriage, terminated employment and/or the potential loss of child, has been identified as a precipitating factor (Meloy, 1998).

As well as increasing the risk of harm to others, including intimates (both real and imagined), insecure attachments are linked to suicide. According to Mecke: 'The facts are incontrovertible. We will never know the reasons for many suicides, but it is undeniable that some persons kill themselves because they become trapped in ill-fated attachments' (2004: ix). What is equally clear is the importance of developmental pathways, with suggestions that: 'The way individuals develop, how they come to see themselves as individuals, and the roles they adopt throughout the maturation process, may have a greater effect on lifetime suicidality than any other factor' (Ledgerwood, 1999: 65). Freud and Bowlby both attended to the subject of suicide and both identified family functioning as a critical factor.[5] For Freud suicide is the product of aggression targeted at a love object turned back against the self (1920: 162):

> Probably no one finds the mental energy required to kill himself unless, in the first place, in doing so he is at the same time killing

---

[5]The relationship between attachment theory and psychoanalysis has not traditionally been an easy one, but hostility and indifference have increasingly given way to cooperation and integration (Holmes, 2001; Fonagy *et al.*, 2008). As a member of the British psychoanalytic movement, Bowlby initially hoped to bring together the competing factions based around Anna Freud, Sigmund's daughter, and Melanie Klein, but only succeeded in uniting them in opposition to his ideas (Holmes, 1993). Despite sharing considerable common ground, attachment theory was rejected by proponents of psychoanalysis and object relations theory for what seem, in retrospect, to have been fairly minor differences of emphasis: Bowlby relied heavily on empirical findings from observational studies of humans and other animals, insisting that children's real life experiences, rather than just their fantasies, are an important source of trauma and gave primacy to a biologically-based need for social relationships rather than to feeding or sexual motives (Rutter, 2008). For these reasons Bowlby was effectively exiled from the psychoanalytic movement. With clarification and some shifts in thinking, however, positions have softened and there is an emerging consensus that attachment theory and psychoanalysis offer complimentary perspectives, which can, and perhaps, should be integrated.

an object with whom he has identified himself, and, in the second place, is turning against himself a death-wish which had been directed against someone else.

The relationship between the suicidal person and the object of his or her intense attachment is said to be characterised by enmeshment in which the suicidal person feels a great deal of ambivalence – they simultaneously love and hate the person (Ledgerwood, 1999). Youth suicide may be triggered by an immediate frustration, but the long-term history typically indicates an increasing inability to cope with rage directed towards parents (Hendin, 1991). Freudian psychoanalysis identifies two processes that lead to suicide: first, the suicidal person seeks to be rid of the attachment figure and suicide provides a means of achieving this; and second, the suicidal person feels an intense guilt or self-blame over their hatred toward someone they care for very much and suicide offers a solution to this dilemma. By killing themselves, the suicidal person has destroyed the attachment with the attachment figure and been punished for his or her transgression against them. Similarly, Bowlby's work has been 'critical to the study of suicide and social relationships' (Ledgerwood, 1999: 67), with several studies having linked suicide to parental loss or abandonment and/or to insecure attachment styles (Adam, 1973; de Jong, 1992; Lyon *et al.*, 2000; Violato and Arato, 2004).

In sum, developmental studies of suicide have identified the following commonalities or themes relating to attachment and individuation: (1) a child-parent relationship characterised by an underlying threat of desertion or taking away love; (2) an underlying ambivalence toward the parent reflecting simultaneous feelings of love and hate with an inability to reconcile the two and a resulting feeling of guilt; (3) the family of the suicidal person is characterised by a profound symbiotic relationship in which he or she must remain faithful only to the family, and normal striving for autonomy and relationships outside the family are seen as disloyal; (4) in this family environment, the suicidal individual fails to pass through the natural stages of psychological development, and has become trapped in a struggle between detachment and enmeshment, leading to suicidal disintegration (Ledgerwood, 1999).

Although firmly focused on individual development, psychoanalysis and attachment theory both contain a social dimension. Freud's work has an 'intrinsically social nature' (Giddens, 1965: 109) and his theory of personality pivots on the relationship between the inner psychic world of the individual and the external world of social reality (Bocock, 2002). Attachment theory also relates directly to social integration, highlighting an essential psycho-social dimension of the social bond (Holmes, 1993; Redman, 2008). What this might mean for the sociology of suicide seems clear: the social conditions that Durkheim and others have pointed to as the 'direct' determinants of the suicide rate cannot be separated from those that influence the development and distribution of personality types in the population. As well as shaping the social circumstances of the potentially suicidal individual, therefore, the currents of egoism and anomie are further implicated in the precipitating conditions of suicide due to their influence on the family and associated patterns of socialisation (Giddens, 1971). Crucially, it has been argued, insecure social conditions produce insecure adults who are, as a result, less able to provide the sort of care that promotes securely attached infants (Holmes, 2001). The key point, then, remains pretty much as it was when Giddens made the following observation more than 40 years ago (1965: 12–13; see also Stack, 1994):

> There are also important empirical lines of convergence between sociological and psychological studies of suicide which offer as yet unexplored research possibilities. Egoistic suicide in Durkheim's conception derives from a low level of integration in social structure. If 'low integration' is considered in terms of the individual member of the group it can be said that it entails the relative detachment of the individual from defined relationships with others. A social structure which is loosely integrated tends to promote the isolation of individuals from closely structured relationships with others…Now one finding which emerges from studies of case-histories of individual suicides is that many suicidal individuals from childhood either (1) show an incapacity to form lasting affective relationships with others, or (2) depend excessively upon one single relationship with another, usually a parent. Here we are evidently approaching the same net result – the social isolation of the individual – from the standpoint of the suicidal personality. The crucial question here is: under what conditions does social

isolation become psychologically 'translated' into a phenomenal situation which the individual defines as 'suicidal'?

The demography of suicide in England and Wales

According to Durkheim the 'suicidal tendency' in European societies grows 'incessantly' from youth to maturity and is much greater, 'often ten times' so, at the close of life than at its beginning (2002: 289):

> The collective force impelling men to kill themselves therefore only gradually penetrates them. All things being equal, they become more accessible to it as they become older, probably because repeated experiences are needed to reveal the complete emptiness of an egoistic life or the total vanity of limitless ambition.

The notion that older people are at a greater risk of suicide than younger people may seem surprising when viewed from our current vantage point and is certainly at odds with the particular concerns that are routinely expressed about the heightened risks facing young men. Press reports have repeatedly drawn attention to the vulnerability of young men in this regard; campaigning organisations have declared suicide to be a major men's health issue; and the government has identified young men as a priority group for action under the various national suicide prevention strategies. The *National Suicide Prevention Strategy for England*, for example, states that 'the majority of suicides now occur in young adult males' (Department of Health, 2002: 7; see also Scottish Executive, 2002).

The heightened rate of young male suicide is often attributed to the uncertainty associated with late modernity and the related 'crisis' of masculinity. Baudelot and Establet (2008: 121), for example, trace the 'new pattern of suicide by age' to the global oil crisis of 1973 and subsequent development of longer, increasingly fragmentary transitions into adulthood. Such trends are said to have 'led to a generalized increase in stress which is reflected in a rise in suicide, attempted suicide (para-suicide), and eating disorders such as anorexia and bulimia' among young people (Furlong and Cartmel, 2007: 87). Much of the discourse surrounding the heightened risks facing young men has drawn on the dominant narrative of gender crisis: that is, of men not knowing how to fit into a changing world in the aftermath of second-wave feminism (Coyle and Morgan-Sykes, 1998). Writing under the headline, *Modern*

Britain is Driving Men to Their Death, Emma Jones, columnist for *The Sun*, a British tabloid newspaper, declared (June 20, 2002):

> It's shocking that the biggest killer of young men in this country is now themselves. The politically correct lobby have undermined men's power and confidence and the feminist pendulum has swung too far. The glory days of manhood, when our grandfathers stood proud in the workshop of the world making steel and building ships are long gone. Men are now more likely to work in an office – jobs which can be done just as well by women. Women enjoy more choice these days – they flit between work and family life with apparent ease. But when men try to counter the balance by taking on traditional female roles, like becoming full time dads, they are laughed at.

What then of the evidence? Looking back over two hundred years, Baudelot and Establet claim that 'the most spectacular of all the transformations to have affected the pattern of suicide' is that concerned with age (2008: 101). Certainly, the general trend across late industrial societies during the final quarter of the twentieth century was one of rising suicide rates among the young and falling rates among older people (Cantor, 2000). In England and Wales, for example, the suicide rate declined among men and women of all ages except men under 45 years, for whom it doubled (Gunnell *et al.*, 2003). The general trend of increasing suicide among young males has recently gone into reverse in many countries (see for example Biddle *et al.*, 2008), but, nonetheless, it remains a leading cause of death within this demographic and youth suicide constitutes the bulk of potential life years lost.

Figure 7.1 shows the number of suicides (and deaths of undetermined intent or 'open verdicts') recorded in England and Wales during 2008 for males and females within various age groups. The trend that is evident is far from linear and young people, by any conventional definition,[6] clearly do not account for the majority of suicides. In terms of raw numbers, the peak age for male suicides is 40–44 years and

---

[6]A key issue here is what we mean by 'young', though it is, of course, not easily resolvable. We suggest however, that people over 40 years of age are not routinely considered to be young and that to refer to young male suicides as including those up to 45 years, as some do, is misleading. The label 'youth' is in fact commonly used to describe the more restricted age range of 16–25 (see, for example the ESRC youth programme, http://www.esrcsocietytoday.ac.uk).

Figure 7.1   Number of Suicides in England and Wales by Age and Sex (2008)

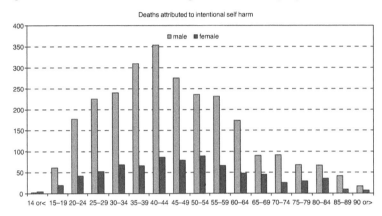

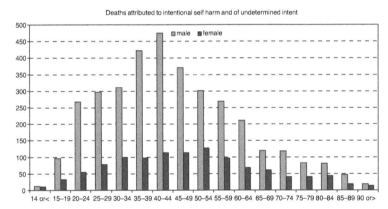

Source: Office for National Statistics (2010a)

suicides among 45–49 year olds outnumber those among 25–29 year olds and 30–34 year olds. Overall, men under the age of 40 account for less than a third of all deaths attributed to intentional self-harm and/or undetermined intent while men under the age of 30 account for no more than one-in-seven of these deaths.[7]

_____

[7]The age distribution of male suicides has changed somewhat in recent years. In 2000, for example, male suicide was more common among 20–29 year olds than 40–49 year olds (Office for National Statistics, 2001). Nonetheless, the peak age for male suicide was 30–35 years and males below the age of 40 accounted for less than a third of all suicides.

Based on these figures we might reasonably conclude that the focus on young people, particularly young men, has diverted attention away from the greater number of suicides among those, particularly men, in mid-life. The raw numbers given here are a poor indicator of risk, however, because they take no account of variations in population size. Adjusting the figures so they represent a rate per 100,000 of population constitutes a much more sensitive measure and further challenges the idea that young men are particularly vulnerable. The suicide rate shown in Figure 7.2 follows a

Figure 7.2   Rate of Suicide in England and Wales per 100,000 by Age and Sex (2008)

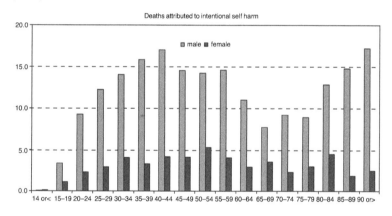

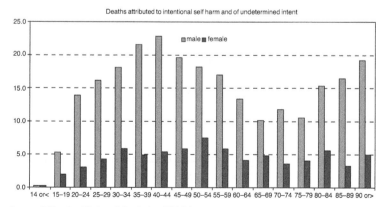

Source: Office for National Statistics (2010a)

bi-modal distribution which indicates that men in mid-life and old-age are at most risk of suicide. Although elderly males account for a relatively small number of suicides, this is largely a result of the mortality rate, which means there are few elderly males in the population, and masks their heightened state of vulnerability. The situation is quite different for older women, with the suicide rate remaining fairly stable over the age of 60 years.

Variations in suicide by age highlight the need for a life-course perspective: we must explain why suicide is relatively unusual among young people, why there is a concentration of suicide among men in mid-life and why older men are also especially vulnerable. What is clear from the outset is that the number of (male) suicides peaks at a significant point in the life-course. A consistent pattern, documented across 72 developed and developing countries, shows that the age distribution of psychological well-being is U-shaped, with happiness typically reaching a low point during mid-life (Blanchflower and Oswald, 2008). National comparisons also indicate that suicide rates and levels of well-being share common predictors, so that higher divorce rates are associated with reduced life satisfaction as well as increased suicide (Helliwell, 2007). In Britain, the peak age for the number of (male) suicides (i.e. 35 to 44 years old) is also the peak age for divorce (ONS, 2010b), while psychological well-being reaches its lowest point among 48 year olds (Blanchflower and Oswald, 2008).

Given that our analysis draws heavily on life-course criminology, it should be noted that suicide differs markedly from crime in terms of its age distribution and, by extension, the implied workings of the social bond. Adolescence represents the peak period of criminal offending, due partly to the relatively weak nature of the social bond during this phase of the life-course. The number of suicides, by contrast, peaks during mid-life, which, we shall argue, reflects the fragmentation of established social bonds. Mid-life stands out as a period of particularly intense investment in work and family life, with the result that it carries a particular set of risks. When these investments turn bad and social bonds begin to unravel an acute sense of meaningless and loss may be experienced, from which suicide may seem to offer a viable escape.

Finally, as a signpost for what is to come, various explanations have been offered for why it is that males account for many more suicides than females – approximately three times as many in England and

Wales during 2008. Women in modern societies, it has been argued, are less exposed to situations of potential anomie than men (Giddens, 1971, 2006). Similarly, women's self-identities are said to be less dependent on labour market status than men's and remain much more closely bound up with child-care; women are said to be integrated into a solid core of intergenerational relationships; and to be more used to adversity – all of which helps to 'inure them to the world's harshness' (Baudelot and Establet, 2008: 177; see also Stack, 2000a). Providing some support for such claims, female suicide rates have been found to be less sensitive than male rates to economic fluctuations, to unemployment and labour market inactivity. Alternatively, it has been suggested that the acquired capability to enact lethal self-injury is generally lower among females than males (Joiner, 2005; Van Orden *et al.*, 2008), which would certainly help to explain the commonly observed pattern whereby more women than men attempt suicide but fewer actually kill themselves. Whatever the precise explanation, and it is likely to be a multi-faceted one, our contention is that differences between male and female suicide rates are strongly related to the workings of the social bond.

A sociological autopsy of suicide – The local picture

Our detailed analysis of 100 case files drawn from a single coroner's office provided for a more thorough investigation of the way that suicide varies with the life-course. The age and sex profiles of these cases were broadly consistent with national figures: male suicides outnumbered female suicides by slightly less than four-to-one and average age at the time of death was 46 years – 44 years for males and 53 years for females. There may be, as Durkheim claimed (2002), nothing that cannot serve as an occasion for suicide, but it is clear from these cases that some things are implicated much more frequently than others and that the meanings and implied aetiological structures vary with the conditions and characteristics of the suicidal individual.

The social circumstances of suicide

The files identified various issues relating to a number of overlapping themes, which included family and interpersonal relationships, work and finance, physical and mental health, drugs and alcohol, intrapersonal distress and crime. In general, the issues that were most frequently cited were those that had to do with family and interpersonal relationships and signs of intrapersonal distress (see Table 7.1). Slightly more than half the cases mentioned relationship problems or breakdown and a third indicated that these difficulties were the main trigger for suicide. The most commonly identified relationship triggers were linked to sexual jealousy and over-dependence, followed by punishment/revenge and disputes over children, with two cases of attempted murder (see below under the heading 'A focus on gender and relationship breakdown'). In addition to these relationship difficulties, problems with children, bereavement and isolation were quite widely cited as were childhood experiences.

The prominence of relationship breakdown and difficulties can be readily explained by attachment theory. Separation from long-term

Table 7.1   Family and Interpersonal Relationships
(percentage of cases where such issues were identified)

Relationship breakdown or difficulties	55
Relationship breakdown etc as trigger	
Breakdown etc identified as main trigger	34
Breakdown etc identified as contributory factors	10
Breakdown etc but not seem to be a trigger	8
Breakdown etc but unclear if a trigger	3
No evidence of breakdown etc	45
Type of trigger	
Sexual jealousy	11
Over-dependence	7
Punishment/revenge	5
Disputes over children	5
Attempted murder	2
Relationship breakdown not cited as main trigger	66
Problems related to children	32
Bereavement	23
Isolation	21
Childhood experiences	17

relationships and divorce are, after all, 'among the most significant of all life events' because they involve the disruption of 'one of the strongest affectional bonds formed by adults' and this disruption is compounded by its 'far reaching implications' (Feeney and Monin, 2008: 934). Attachment theory also helps to explain why reactions to separation and divorce vary in the way they do, predicting that traumatic life events are most stressful for individuals with troubled attachment histories and insecure attachment orientations. Such individuals are said to be particularly prone to break down after loss or separation because the separation 'confirms their worst fears and expectations' and is likely to reactivate earlier unresolved separations from attachment figures (Feeney and Monin, 2008: 941). What this means in cases of suicide is that relationship breakdown is generally considered to be a precipitating factor or trigger, which operates on the basis of an underlying vulnerability or predisposing factor that is rooted in an insecure attachment style. The vulnerabilities that come with insecure attachments are further evident from cases where childhood experiences were implicated: these experiences included things such as physical and/or sexual abuse, neglect and separation, all of which make it extremely unlikely that a secure base will be established.

The signs of intrapersonal distress that were most widely cited were those relating to mental health, suicide history and substance use. Approximately three-fifths (61 per cent) of cases identified depression or some other mental health diagnosis, with slightly less than half (45 per cent) citing use of anti-depressants. Almost two-fifths (38 per cent) noted previous suicide attempts and a further one-in-ten (9 per cent) mentioned previous threats of suicide. A quarter (24 per cent) mentioned drug and/or alcohol dependence, with slightly less than a fifth (16 per cent) identifying alcohol and/or drug use at the time of death. In addition to these issues, physical health problems (38 per cent), criminal offending (21 per cent), employment issues (20 per cent) and childhood experiences (17 per cent) were cited quite widely. Much less commonly mentioned were debt (10 per cent), shame (9 per cent) and crime victimisation (8 per cent).

The social context of suicide across the life-course
Further analysis indicated that the social circumstances surrounding suicide varied quite markedly according to the age and sex of the

Table 7.2   How the Social Circumstances of Suicide Vary by Age and Sex (Cramer's V)

	Age	Sex
Family and interpersonal relationships		
Relationship breakdown	0.42*	0.03
Relationship breakdown as trigger	0.29*	0.20
Relationship breakdown – type of trigger	0.38	0.51
Problems related to children	0.36*	0.28*
Bereavement	0.29	0.03
Isolation	0.25	0.28*
Childhood experiences	0.48*	0.03
Signs of intrapersonal distress		
Depression or mental health diagnosis	0.26	0.21*
Anti-depressants	0.34*	0.13
Suicide history	0.25	0.20
Alcohol and/or drug dependency	0.26	0.06
Alcohol and/or drugs at time of suicide	0.31	0.02
Work and finance		
Employment	0.38*	0.14
Debt	0.18	0.09
Other		
Physical health	0.56*	0.15
Crime – perpetrator	0.28	0.27*
Crime – victim	0.30	0.03
Shame	0.20	0.16

$* = p < .05$
Note:
i.   Age was divided into the following bands: 16 to 24 years, 25 to 34 years, 35 to 44 years, 45 to 54 years and 55 to 64 years.
ii. The relationships shown here were principally assessed on the basis of Cramer's V, which indicates the strength of association between the relevant variables. This statistic was used, rather than one specially designed for ordinal variables, because we did not want to make any assumptions about the nature of the relationships involved (e.g. that they are linear-like) and because we wanted to compare the relations involving age with those involving sex.
iii. Probability values were used as a secondary indicator even though the data did not meet the assumption of being based on a random sample drawn from a wider population.

victim. On the whole, such circumstances were associated more strongly with age than sex, though there were one or two exceptions to this general pattern (see Table 7.2). Age was most strongly linked to physical health and childhood experiences, followed by relationship breakdown, problems with children and work-related issues. The variations that were evident in this regard pointed towards three distinct aetiological structures – young people in crisis, mid-life gendered patterns of work and family and older people in decline.

1) Young people in crisis

Adolescence has traditionally been viewed as a period of 'storm and stress', but this characterisation has increasingly been challenged on the grounds that it is unsupported by evidence (Coleman and Hendry, 1999). Repeated studies have shown that a minority of young people experience a turbulent adolescence and that the majority manage the transition reasonably well. This is not to deny that adolescence is a period of significant change, nor that these changes may create a heightened sense of insecurity and vulnerability, but they do not ordinarily result in suicidal behaviour. Although suicidal thoughts are not uncommon, relatively few young people try to kill themselves, with recent British research suggesting a figure of 5 per cent among 16–24 year olds (Meltzer *et al.*, 2002). Far from being an ordinary feature of adolescent development, suicidal behaviour among young people has been found to follow a suicidal career or 'pathways' model, whereby it is typically associated with a long history of disturbed behaviour and very negative relationships with parents (Maris, 1981; Stack, 2000b). Family problems, including loss of parent(s) and disturbed or insecure attachments in childhood have been widely implicated in meta-analyses of adolescent suicide (Violato and Arato, 2004), while suicide attempts and serious suicidal ideation among young people have been linked to the perceived absence of parents as emotionally available attachment figures (de Jong, 1992; see also Lyon *et al.*, 2000).

The role of attachments is also apparent from evidence that the creation of secure attachments with parents, extra familial adults and/or peers is pivotal to young people's healing from suicidal feelings (Bostik and Everall, 2007). A secure attachment is said to bring many benefits in this context, including improved self-perceptions, an increased sense of hope and self-worth and the promotion of reliable support systems. Such evidence is consistent with earlier findings that people who attempt suicide are considerably less isolated than are those who actually kill themselves (Stengel, 1958) as well as more recent findings that social contact helps to explain why some groups are less prone to suicide than others (Baudelot and Establet, 2008).

Our results are consistent with the notion that adolescent suicide is associated with a particular sense of crisis and damaged family attachments. What was most distinctive about the cases involving young people under the age of 25 years was the extent to which they were linked with negative childhood experiences and previous suicide attempts. Childhood experiences were cited in three-fifths (60 per cent) of such cases compared with approximately one-in-ten (12 per cent) cases involving older people. The relative infrequency with which childhood experiences were implicated among older adults may not be a reliable indicator of actual experience, however, and may simply reflect a tendency in the files to concentrate on precipitating factors as the most proximate 'cause'. Although the association between age and previous suicide history appeared to be fairly modest, the overall figure masked some notable differences between young people and older adults: all but one of the cases involving young people under the age of 25 years mentioned previous suicide attempts or threats compared with less than half of those involving older adults.

2)   *Mid-life gendered patterns*

Suicides in mid-life were found to be associated with an appreciably different set of circumstances, which reflected the changing roles and responsibilities associated with the life-course, while also highlighting the contingent nature of what are often thought of as protective factors. Numerous studies within criminology and suicidology have highlighted the protective value of the social bond, particularly in the form of work and family life. When these aspects of life are functioning well they serve to give people a sense of purpose and belonging, but when they begin to unravel they may stop being a source of protection and become a source of risk. Work-related problems, particularly in the form of redundancy and unemployment, and family breakdown are known to be associated with suicidal behaviour (Platt and Hawton, 2000; Stack, 2000) and were widely implicated among our cases where the victim was in mid-life. Work-related problems were cited in approximately one-in-three (35 per cent) cases where the victim was aged between 35 and 64 years, but in no more than one-in-six cases outside of this age-range. Relationship breakdown was most widely cited where the victim was between 16 and 54 years old and was most widely implicated as a main trigger where they were 25 to 54 years old (see Table 7.3). Young adults are clearly not immune from relationship breakdown or the associated emotional fall-out, but, broadly speaking, they are likely to be less invested in the permanence of their relationship than older adults, so that its breakdown is less likely to trigger suicide. This explanation is certainly consistent with, and helps to explain, the concentration of suicide among those in mid-life. Similarly, problems with children were most commonly identified where the victim was between 25 and 54 years old.

Table 7.3 Relationship Breakdown and Problems Related to Children by Age (percentages)

	Relationship breakdown	Relationship breakdown ...		Problems related to children
		main trigger	contributory factor	
Age in years				
16–24	60	20	10	30
25–34	81	57	10	52
35–44	59	47	12	41
45–54	65	35	20	40
55–64	43	29	7	14
65 or above	18	6	0	6

The role of work and family problems was mediated by gender. To some extent, male vulnerability seemed to be linked to threats to the traditional provider role: work-related problems and debt were cited at twice the rate for males as females (23 per cent compared with 10 per cent and 11 per cent compared with 5 per cent respectively). Gender roles were further implicated in regard to family life. Relationship breakdown was cited at a very similar rate regardless of the sex of the victim, but was more likely to be identified as the main trigger for males. Among male victims, relationship breakdown tended to be identified as the main trigger rather than as a contributory factor (38 per cent compared with 9 per cent), whereas female victims were more evenly divided between these two categories

(19 per cent and 14 per cent respectively). Female suicides were further distinguished by the extent to which they were more widely associated with problems related to children (57 per cent of females compared with 25 per cent of males). Such problems included separation from children due to divorce, estrangement (especially from older children) and children being taken into care. While male suicides tended to be associated with relationship breakdown in the absence of problems related to children (30 per cent of males compared with 10 per cent of females), female suicides tended to be associated with relationship breakdown and problems related to children (43 per cent of females compared with 25 per cent of males) or problems related to children in the absence of relationship breakdown (14 per cent and none respectively).[8]

What are we to make of such differences? Women may be better able to manage relationship breakdown (Cantor, 2000), particularly when their role as mothers remains intact. At the same time, it is worth noting that relationship breakdown may tend to mean different things for men and women. If Durkheim was right and feminist critiques of traditional marriage are well-founded, women will be more likely than men to see separation as freeing them from an unhappy situation. Also, given prevailing social and legal norms, separation and divorce routinely distances men from their children in a way that it rarely does for women. For such men relationship breakdown cannot be easily separated from their role as parents because it tends to limit their involvement in family life more generally (Owen, 2003). Under these circumstances, separation and divorce can be seen to challenge men's role as fathers and, by extension, their sense of belonging and purpose even when there are no manifest problems relating to their children: that is to say, relationship breakdown may represent a challenge to fatherhood even if this challenge remains latent and implicit. Whatever the precise explanation, family breakdown poses a serious threat to the social bond for both men and women and is a key antecedent of suicide during mid-life, hence we return to it later in the chapter for more developed qualitative analysis.

---

[8]For family breakdown (combining relationship breakdown and problems related to children) by sex, Cramer's V = 0.4, p < .05.

Other notable sex differences were evident in relation to mental health, experiences of isolation and crime victimisation. Depression or some other mental health diagnosis was more commonly cited in relation to female than male suicides (80 per cent compared with 56 per cent) as was a sense of isolation (43 per cent compared with 15 per cent). None of the female cases, compared with one-in-four (27 per cent) of the male cases mentioned criminal behaviour.

3) Older people in decline

As with much previous research our findings suggest that the antecedents of suicide are different for the elderly than for younger and middle-age groups. Suicide among older people is less closely associated with interpersonal and relationship problems, financial, legal and occupational difficulties and more closely associated with physical illness and other losses (see also Cattell, 2000). Our analysis shows that the extent to which physical health problems were cited increased sharply with age (see Figure 7.3). Differences regarding mental health were much less marked and rather more ambiguous, while references to anti-depressants did not vary greatly by age (except they were rarely cited in cases involving 16–24 year olds). Notable differences were evident in relation to bereavement, however, which was cited in almost half the cases involving older people

Figure 7.3   Health Status by Age (percentage)

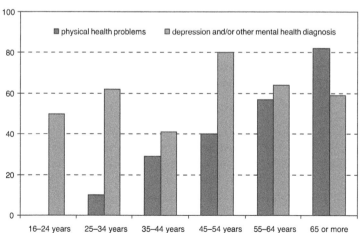

(47 per cent of those aged 65 years or above compared with 18 per cent of those in younger groups). Surprisingly, perhaps, this did not translate into a particular emphasis on the isolation of older victims: the differences that were evident in this regard were relatively minor and did not form a clear or coherent pattern. Nonetheless, bereavement and physical decline may be understood in terms of a weakened social bond as they reflect a loss of emotional attachment and potentially compromised social participation.

Drug and alcohol issues were rarely cited in cases involving people over the age of 64 years and, to a lesser extent, between 55–64 years. Other than this, variations by age were either minor or did not form a clear or coherent pattern.

A focus on gender and relationship breakdown

At this point we further develop our analysis of gendered contexts of relationship breakdown and suicide, with reference to the qualitative data. This section of the chapter illustrates the kinds of distinctive insights that a qualitative approach to suicide research can bring. As noted above (under 'mid-life gendered patterns'), relationship breakdown suicides are especially pertinent to those aged 25 years and over and to men (at least as a main trigger). In categorising those suicides (n=34) where relationship breakdown seemed to be the main trigger we had regard to the apparent response of the suicidal individual to the relationship problems (or relationship termination in many cases). The response categories we identified were murder/attempted murder, punishment, dependence, sexual jealousy and separation from children. It should be noted that these are, of course, not discrete categories. 'Punishment' cases tended to also involve sexual jealousy and/or separation from children, for example. The typology is simply designed to highlight the dominant circumstances as suggested by the evidence presented to the coroner. With the exception of one woman, all such cases involved the breakdown of heterosexual relationships.

Most of what follows applies to men's suicides, as only four of the 34 suicides where relationship breakdown was thought to be the principal trigger were women. Particular caution is needed in drawing any conclusions about women's suicides in the light of the very small number of cases included here. Nonetheless, for women, the context of the relationship breakdown was most commonly categorised as over-dependence whereas for males it was more likely to be sexual jealousy, punishment/revenge or disputes over children. Of the four women where relationship breakdown was cited as the main trigger, three were categorised as cases of over-dependence and the other as sexual jealousy. Therefore, punishment/revenge, disputes over children and murder/attempted murder were identified as the main trigger for male suicides only. Again, caution is needed because some sub-categories within the typology of circumstances are based on very small numbers of cases (sometimes five or less).

Drawing on a psychoanalytic framework, Giddens (1971) argues that suicide has various unconscious or semi-conscious symbolic meanings where death is not treated simply as an end to existence. Death through suicide, he maintains, can be invested with instrumental significance, either as a 'magical' solution to problems or as a weapon to secure a desired end. As such, suicide 'is in an inverted way an attempt at *mastery*: an attempt to control and rectify an intolerable state of affairs': the victim's 'world has slipped away from him, and yet in the very act of denying that world he attempts to encompass and change it as well as to change himself' (Giddens, 1971: 113). Among the meanings and attempts at mastery that are identified, Giddens draws attention to the following: 1) 'Retaliatory abandonment': a person who has, or considers themselves to have been, abandoned by a friend or loved one takes their own life in an act of retaliation, thus abandoning the person who has abandoned them; 2) Reunion: suicide offers a way of reuniting with a loved one who has died or left; 3) Revenge: suicide is an aggressive act against another who has 'wronged' the suicidal individual; 4) Rebirth: suicide is a means of changing identity, of being born anew. While similar themes are identified by Douglas (1967), Giddens makes it clear that these meanings are rooted in the social condition of the suicidal individual: the essential point linking social and psychological factors in egoistic suicide, he argues, 'can therefore be said to be in the reciprocal "push" towards the *isolation of the suicidal individual from relationships that are significant to him and on which he is highly dependent*' (1971: 108, original emphasis). As such, '*egoistic suicide represents an expiatory attempt at or appeal for reintegration within a relationship or a group*', though the meanings, particularly the degree of externalised aggression involved, will vary depending on whether 'revenge', 'retaliatory abandonment' or 'reunion' provide the dominant motif (1971: 109, original emphasis). What we would like to add is that these meanings and motifs are bound up with gendered discourses of power and control.

1)   Murder and attempted murder

The theme of mastery is dramatically illustrated by (attempted) murder-suicides. Reconsider the case of Brian Philcox, for example, with which we began this chapter: 'forced' into a divorce he did not want and left 'frustrated at every turn' and 'completely broken' by his attempts to negotiate access to his children, Philcox was reported to have been overheard by a neighbour saying: 'I have lost my wife. I have lost my kids. I am going to lose my house. They can all f*** off. I would rather burn the house than give it to that bitch'. Of our 100 cases, two involved (attempted) murder-suicides and, typically, both were male: 85 per cent of murder-suicide suspects in Barraclough and Harris's (2002) study of all such cases in England and Wales from 1998 to 1992 were men. One of the cases we studied was a multiple murder of wife and children, in the context of depression and major debts, but apparently no history of violence. The other was a case with multiple long-term problems, including alcohol problems and domestic violence as well as the recent death (possibly suicide) of a teenage son. The victim of the attempted murder was the man's wife, who was left for dead, though she survived with serious impairment. He killed himself on the assumption she was dead, saying he 'couldn't face prison' and wanted to be reunited with his dead son.

2)   Punishment

The themes of revenge and retaliatory abandonment were evident in a series of cases, which gave an impression of men to whom control of a woman partner was all-important: so important, perhaps, that the inability to control her in life could lead to the extreme gesture of self-destruction. Or rather to a desire to control beyond death, as can be seen vividly in Case 7. Here a note was left by a man who specifically addressed his ex-partner's anticipated guilt following his suicide:

> How do you deal with things knowing Lewis's dad killed himself because of you? All those times he looked at you lovingly and you killed his dad. (Case 7, excerpt from suicide note)

In another case (no. 66) the entire suicide note read 'Congratulations. You win.' These cases can be usefully understood in the context of

other evidence of some men's preoccupation with control in intimate relationships. The obvious reference point here is feminist work
on domestic abuse which has emphasised tactics of control along a
continuum of physically and emotionally abusive behaviour (Dobash
and Dobash, 1979) and has argued that for men to seek to control in
intimate relationships is relatively mainstream.

3)   Over-dependence

The idea of dependence on a partner is a more traditional gendered
narrative for women than for men. Over-dependence did feature for
three of the four women in our sample whose suicides were considered to be primarily triggered by relationship breakdown. One such
example was of a woman who had multiple problems, but seemed
to be prompted to suicide by over-dependence on an ex-long-term
woman partner whose surname she had taken as if in marriage.
She had split up with a more recent girlfriend because she still had
feelings for her ex-partner and then killed herself soon afterwards.
Four of the male suicides in the sample were put in the dependence
category. One man wrote in his suicide note that:

> Going out is the only way I can cope with things. I'm not looking
> for anyone else. You're in my head all of the time. (Case 83, excerpt
> from suicide note)

We could speculate that for men there are, perhaps, tensions between
the ideal of autonomy that hegemonic masculinity sets up and the
reality of dependence on women, which results in distress. Distress
may also be caused by a tension between certain misogynist aspects
of heterosexual male culture and the personal experience of depending
on a real embodied woman. The dependence for men can of course
be material as well as emotional (McMahon, 1999) and the language
of dependence can also be a subtle tactic of control. Caught in an
apparently unresolvable situation, suicide may come to be seen as
a 'magical' solution offering release or, as indicated in the previous
quote, providing a means of coping.

4)   Sexual jealousy

Eleven cases, ten of them involving men, seem to have been primarily
characterised by sexual jealousy although control and revenge would

again seem to be key themes within this category. Proprietorial sexuality is an important aspect of hegemonic masculinity. There are often strong overtones of shame and dishonour in these cases, where the distress may, perhaps, have as much to do with being *seen* to be betrayed by a partner as the 'betrayal' itself. Below are excerpts from the case files where sexual jealousy seemed to be the principal context of the suicidal act.

> He came to my door covered in blood. He said 'she's ripped my heart out, she's thrown it on the floor and she's bouncing on it'. He was so upset, he also said 'she's shagging someone in the bed I paid for'. (Case 40 – mother's statement to police)

> SO YOU NOT SEEING ANYONE ELSE, I JUST SAW YOU BOTH. HOPE YOU HAPPY I WILL BE WHERE I'M GOING GOODBYE. REMEMBER I LOVED YOU YEAH. (Case 50 [male] – excerpt from mobile phone records)

As well as the themes of blame, jealousy, revenge and, potentially, retaliatory abandonment and an imagined reunion, the second of these quotes conveys a sense of omnipotence that was frequently in evidence. According to Freud (1953), the unconscious does not believe in its own death and acts as if it is immortal. In the second of these quotes the suicidal individual seems to be imagining a life beyond death – a rebirth perhaps – by encouraging his ex-partner to remember him as somebody who loved her.

5)   *Separation from children*

Although problems related to children were significantly associated with women's suicides in our sample, none of the women's suicides which we categorised as *primarily* triggered by relationship breakdown featured separation from children as a core issue. All these cases involved men and in some the suicidal act seemed to be imbued with the qualities of a 'magical' solution, offering a way of ending the pains of separation:

> I've lost everything and ain't got no contact with my son or family phone number ... I love and miss Nicholas David I love

and miss and can't go on with the heartache. (Case 19 – excerpt from suicide note)

He hasn't seen his two children for a few months now, Rachel 6 and Jack 5. Not seeing his children has broken his heart....Joe has told me that he wanted to kill himself because of his children. (Case 23 – excerpt from mother's statement to the police)

We might speculate that in a climate where involved fatherhood has fairly recently developed a certain cultural status (even if men's actual practices may be mixed), hegemonic masculinity could perhaps be seen to be shifting so that inability to fulfil involved fatherhood because of relationship breakdown might seem as much of a challenge as losing the breadwinner role would have done in earlier times. At the same time, the theme of emotional loss remains a core one. For both men and women, when adult intimate relationships are so fluid, children may take on a new significance (Beck and Beck-Gernsheim, 1995: 37):

The child becomes the last remaining, irrevocable, unique primary love object. Partners come and go, but the child stays ...The child becomes the final alternative to loneliness, a bastion against the vanishing chances of loving and being loved.

In addition, the inevitable gap between the raised expectations of the 'pure relationship' in late modernity (Giddens, 1992) and the mundane reality of relationship conflict can cause unhappiness. Perhaps these influences do not affect men and women in the same way. An important part of the cultural context is the angry politics of fatherhood, with fathers' rights organisations using stories of suicide to bolster their campaigns against the Child Support Agency and/or the family courts.

So, if we re-examine the suicides that are primarily triggered by relationship breakdown, gender differences are very apparent. If we regard homicidal violence, punishment, sexual jealousy and conflict over children as signifying different aspects of domestic abuse, then 23 suicides (all of them men) out of the sample of 100 would come under this heading. There is, of course, a risk that a focus on abusiveness might pathologise these men and we should bear in mind that their extreme actions may be understood as illegitimate attempts to achieve legitimate human goods such as security, mastery and a sense of belonging (see Ward and Maruna, 2007).

Conclusion

Some of what we have presented above, especially in the more quantitatively-oriented section of the chapter, is fairly familiar from epidemiological research, though we have challenged the conventional wisdom that young men are particularly at risk of suicide by highlighting the large number of suicides recorded among those in mid-life and the particular vulnerability of elderly men. Beyond this the chapter makes a contribution to the study of suicide in two respects. Firstly, it begins to demonstrate the potential of qualitative and mixed methods research – the sociological autopsy – within a field traditionally dominated by quantitative methods. Secondly, it has sought to develop a more fully theorised account by drawing on criminological work which emphasises the role of the social bond across the life-course. Although the link between suicide and social integration has been well-established, differentiation of this across the life-course is less well examined. Studies of crime and suicide provide ample evidence of the importance of the protective value of the social bond, particularly in the form of work and personal attachments. But the flip side of this protective role means that when work and family life come under strain they may become a source of tension rather than support, of risk rather than protection.

Although the weakening of the social bond seems to play an important role, we recognise that it does not fully explain incidence of suicide, not least because many people negotiate the vicissitudes of life without killing themselves. Piecing together the evidence suggests that suicide may be usefully understood as the result of an interaction between social (contextual) and psychological (personal) risks and between predisposing and precipitating factors. Or, put another way, as the result of 'a combination of (psychiatric) vulnerability, situational stress and individual perceptions' (Liebling, 1992: 85). Attachment theory has much to offer in this regard because the essential link between social and psychological factors in many suicides seems to be a 'push' towards the isolation of the individual from significant relationships and because the theory allows for the accumulation of distal and prox-

imal influences. We must be careful not to apply the theory in a mech-
anistic or deterministic way, however, because, as Laub and Sampson
(2003) emphasise, any attempt to theorise the life-course should allow
for its essential malleability. While attachment styles can and do adapt,
a certain degree of stability is, nonetheless, evident and this helps to
explain why people react differently to apparently similar conditions.
The meaning of separation and divorce, for example, varies because
people's 'working models' differ. For those with an insecure attachment style, the bonds they manage to create, linking them to jobs,
partners and children may assume such great importance, as the only
form of security they have known, that their loss, or even its possibility, is unbearable. It is in this context, perhaps, that the loss of one's
home becomes potentially suicidogenic (Stack and Wasserman, 2007).

The workings of the social bond are relevant to each of the aetiological structures we have identified – young people in crisis, mid-
life gendered patterns of work and family and older people in decline.
They also help to explain both the large number of suicides among
men in mid-life and the particular vulnerability of the elderly. Family
problems, including loss and disturbed or insecure attachments in
childhood, are widely implicated in the suicides of young people,
while the prominence of bereavement and physical decline in suicides
of the elderly can also potentially be understood in terms of a weakened social bond. Bereavement involves a loss of personal attachments
while physical incapacity compromises the potential for social participation, reinforcing the sense that there is nothing to live for. Among
those in mid-life, the workings of the social bond are different again
as this is a period of particularly intense investment in work and
family life. Comparisons with adolescence are especially telling here,
in part, at least, because of the way in which such investments are
built up over time.

Although often characterised as a time of upheaval and vulnerability,
'storm and stress' models of adolescence tend to exaggerate the volatil-
ity of this phase of the life-course. Young people are generally less
socially embedded than at any other time, but this is a largely normative experience, whereby a certain distancing from family of origin
is considered part and parcel of growing up. Weakened social bonds
during mid-life, on the other hand, carry a rather different set of meanings and convey a sharper sense of loss and personal failure. By their
mid-to-late-30s, most people have begun to accumulate a considerable

investment in work and family life and this investment is likely to be central to their sense of self and to their place in the world, making them particularly vulnerable when these things come under threat. It is in this context, perhaps, that Raoul Moat's comments about having lost everything and being too old to rebuild his life should be understood. The role of the social bond also helps to explain why so many more men than women kill themselves. Traditional expectations about the male provider role may mean that work-related problems and financial difficulties strike a particularly profound blow to men's sense of purpose and belonging. Added to this, the relatively fragile position of fatherhood means that relationship breakdown tends to come with an added cost for men – one that serves to undermine their sense of attachment and involvement. While women may be better able to manage relationship breakdown, their role as mothers also provides a protected attachment and a relatively robust social bond. The importance of family dynamics is clearly evident from the way in which suicide appears to be bound up with the angry politics of fatherhood, with jealousy, control and with domestic relationships that may be considered abusive.

Finally, the workings of the social bond can, and perhaps should, be related to the conditions of anomie and egoism. Whilst it has been suggested elsewhere that men are particularly exposed to situations of potential anomie because their roles and identities are more tightly bound up with work and public life (Giddens, 1971 and 2006), we can go further than this. We can say that men in mid-life are highly exposed to the possibility of anomic-failure and egoistic-loss: their heavy investment in work and family life poses a particular set of risks in both spheres and the deprivations of divorce, separation and family breakdown are not only at their height during this stage of the life-course, but weigh particularly heavily on men. Suicides among younger and older people seem, by comparison, to be tipped towards the egoistic rather than the anomic. Young people do have to negotiate many situations where the potential for anomic-failure is high, but such situations are rarely implicated in their suicide: the impact of failure is, perhaps, generally off-set by a future orientation which offers hope and the possibility of recovery. The prominence of attachment-related issues in cases involving young people, with all the implications of emotional isolation, is primarily suggestive of egoistic suicide. Suicide in later life, it has been suggested, is more ambiguous because older people tend to be isolated from regular ties with others, but are also placed, quite suddenly, in a position where they no longer feel themselves to be useful members of society (Giddens, 1971). The evidence presented in this chapter helps to clarify such matters. If status frustration were the primary driver of suicide among older people we would expect to see a marked increase in and around the retirement age, but we do not: the suicide rate among men follows a downward curve through the sixties, levelling off in the seventies, before increasing markedly during the eighties and nineties. Far from suggesting status frustration, the downturn in the suicide rate among men in their sixties and seventies, coinciding as it does with a general upturn in psychological well-being, supports the suggestion that, having learnt to adapt to their strengths and weaknesses, older people have quelled their 'infeasible aspirations' (Blanchflower and Oswald, 2008: 1747). Added to this, the pattern of physical decline and bereavement associated with older suicides seems more egoistic than anomic, implying a loss of meaningful attachments and of life turning in on itself.

8
Lessons for Prevention

Our aim in writing this book was to disseminate both the method and the findings of the sociological autopsy study. We begin this final chapter by summarising what we see as the book's contribution and then we address the question of suicide prevention, including the ways in which our sociological autopsy study can potentially inform prevention.

The book's contribution

We are not the first to try and work with dual paradigms in social research. Hammersley (1992) has coined the term 'subtle realism' and Bhaskar 'critical realism' to convey the idea that researchers can convey truths about social phenomena whilst also maintaining a critical perspective on the constructed nature of the available evidence.[9] Although there are methodological writings such as these which touch on the possibility of operating dual paradigms, it is perhaps not so usual for social scientists to publish developed empirical examples of dual paradigm research, so we would claim to be making a valuable contribution to sociology in this regard. More clearly, however, we are attempting to bring new life to the sociological study of

---

[9]These two differ in political orientation, with Bhaskar stressing the role of research in social critique and emancipation, whereas Hammersley emphasises the researcher's responsibility to avoid politicisation of the research process, arguing for a 'nonfoundationalist realism' (Hammersley and Gomm, 1997).

suicide specifically, a field where arguments raged about epistemology and ontology some decades ago but where things have gone
rather quiet more recently and where most research is exclusively quantitative and positivist in orientation. We hope our study demonstrates the utility of a qualitatively-driven mixed methods approach
to the study of suicide. We also have sought to illustrate the value of
sociological research on individual suicide cases. Whilst not rejecting insights from other disciplines, we have emphasised the sociological contribution to case-based research, as these kinds of studies
tend in practice to take a predominantly psychiatric focus and
psycho-social approaches are rare.

Our over-arching aim has been to reinvigorate the sociology of
suicide by moving out of the shadow cast by Durkheim. This we
have sought to do by transcending the core sociological dichotomies
that imbued his work and that of others who followed in its wake.
Rejecting the separations and divisions that are all too common
within sociology, we have provided a double reading of suicide that
draws on both constructionist and objectivist traditions. Over the
course of the empirical chapters we moved from a constructivist perspective to a more objectivist one. Chapters 4 and 5 were broadly constructionist discussions of the nature of evidence in coroners' files.
Chapter 6 was a bridging chapter which moved towards a more objectivist stance via a thick description of the social meanings on suicidal
actions. Chapter 7 was then more firmly in an objectivist tradition,
presenting bivariate analysis of the statistical profile of the 100 suicides
and making theoretical connections with the idea of the social bond
across the life-course. This quantitative focus was, however, followed
by a return to qualitative detail, in relation to a specific theme, re-
emphasising the importance of social meanings. The double reading
we have provided points to both interpretive and structural dimensions of suicide and, drawing these dimensions together, we have suggested that such behaviour may be usefully thought of as a form
of structured action. The causes of suicide are, ultimately, to be found
in the meanings and motivations of individuals, but this does not
provide a complete explanation as it ignores the regularities and patterns that can be found in incidence of suicide. As we have shown
in Chapters 6 and 7, suicide and its attendant meanings are structured
by the life-course. More than this, we contend that structures and
meanings are mutually reinforcing, so that suicide may usefully be

understood as a form of reproduced practice: a person incorporates suicide within their repertoire of action in response to the cluster of circumstances that they find themselves in and, by taking their own life, they reinforce the idea that suicide is a viable response to such circumstances. This process helps to explain cases where a husband kills himself in a similar way and in similar circumstances to his wife several years after her death (see Chapter 6). By extension, approaching suicide as a form of reproduced practice may offer useful insights into apparent suicide clusters such as those that have recently been documented in Bridgend and Belfast (*The Observer*, January 27, 2008; *Belfast Telegraph*, October 21 2010). In line with Giddens' (1984) theory of structuration, we suggest that 'agential processes' work reciprocally with situations and structures, insofar as situations and structures are partly determined by choices made by individuals, and at the same time constrain and modify the choices available to them.

As for our more specific substantive findings, these divide into insights about the construction of evidence about suicides and insights into the aetiology of suicidal acts. In fact we see these two domains as connected, insofar as the stock of knowledge that bereaved family members and professionals have about why someone might kill themselves is similar to the stock of knowledge a distressed individual will draw on in deciding what it is an appropriate response to adversity (as noted above). That said, we have consistently used the term 'dual paradigms' rather than claiming to be mixing or merging ontological paradigms, because constructionism and objectivism do not neatly fit with each other and one does not straightforwardly lead into the other as might be supposed by the structure of our book. A focus on the construction of evidence in coroners' files shows the influence of the concerns of the living on evidence about the dead. We see the concerns of relatives to negotiate the hovering possibility of blame and we see professionals arguing that the death was beyond their control. The dead could acquire new identities in the course of the inquest and these could also be contested. Our study of suicide notes reveals the importance of family and other close social relationships, with a particular focus on the role of apologies in confirming connection or disconnection with significant others. We noted that the primary agency of the notes' authors tends to be muted. The lessons from the constructionist chapters that can be carried forward into a more objectivist approach are the over-riding importance of social relationships in inquest evidence and the fundamentally contested and messy nature of the evidence in coroners' case files. The role of intimate relationships continued to have a high profile in the two chapters (6 and 7) which were more focused on understanding suicidal acts. This analysis highlighted the significance of social bonds such as close relationships and work in making sense of suicide; the importance of a focus on gendered identities and gendered practices; and the potential for attachment theory to provide helpful insights, alongside sociological concepts.

Limitations of our method

It needs to be acknowledged that there are limitations to the sociological autopsy method as we implemented it. We used only coroners' files. These documents can be limited in various ways. As noted in Chapter 3, data on social class are inconsistently recorded and data on ethnicity often absent. The files vary considerably in terms of the amount of evidence and level of detail about social context. The purpose of the inquest is to establish how the death should be categorised and not to establish causal factors. A richer qualitative picture should emerge if interviews were conducted with friends and family, as in the qualitative dimension of Owens *et al.*'s (2008) psychological autopsy study. A more robust quantitative examination could be conducted via a case-control study which perhaps involved living controls with similar levels of mental ill health. A much richer picture of socio-economic circumstances could be achieved if the deceased were geographically located. Both area-based social deprivation and individual social class are important to consider in relation to suicidal behaviour (Platt, 2011). As explained in Chapter 3, we decided on ethical grounds not to record any identifying details such as geographical location or place of death and this decision placed limitations on the kinds of analysis that were possible. There is, however, considerable potential to expand a dual paradigms, mixed method sociological autopsy study beyond the limitations of our study of coroners' files.

Having re-stated what we see as the book's contribution and assessed the limitations of the method, we move on at this point to consider suicide prevention – firstly the evidential basis of current strategies and secondly the potential contribution of our own research approach and its findings to informing suicide prevention.

Preventing suicide

Suicide prevention has risen up the agenda of Western governments in the last couple of decades (Taylor *et al.*, 1997), with suicide rates often viewed as a key indicator of levels of general mental well-being in the population (Gavin and Rogers, 2006). As Wainwright and Calnan (2008) suggest (with reference to the UK) it is only relatively recently that there has been explicit engagement with policies designed to militate against mental ill health as an important part of policies designed to promote general health and well-being. Suicide tends to be conceived in these national strategies as primarily a *health* problem rather than a social problem. Not surprisingly, therefore, the policy engagement with suicide prevention has tended to rest on the same kinds of research evidence as are applied right across the field of health and medicine. As has been suggested in this book and elsewhere, the reliance on psychology and psychiatry in developing strategies for suicide prevention has largely squeezed out other ways of interrogating suicide or making recommendations for suicide prevention (Hjelmeland and Knizek, 2010). Key concerns for the rest of this chapter are to note the methodological approaches which have thus far informed key policies, strategies or recommendations and then reflect on how the findings of the sociological autopsy study may be useful in complimenting the evidence that is already applied to suicide prevention. Insights from our study are not intended to refute the kinds of observations made using other methods or from other disciplinary perspectives but rather to add to them in the spirit of interdisciplinarity.

National suicide prevention strategies

In 1998 Keith Hawton wrote an editorial for the British Medical Journal that provided a rationale for the development and maintenance of suicide prevention strategies. Whilst cautioning against the setting of reduction targets that are not informed by 'hard longitudinal data' (Hawton, 1998: 156), he warns of the dangers of setting unmeasurable targets – using the example of depression as difficult to target due to 'incidence' and 'subsequent disability' as well as problems with reliable measurement. Despite these warnings, Hawton goes on to suggest that effective measurable targets aimed at populations that are known to be high risk are important and that to abandon targets at a time when other countries were establishing suicide prevention strategies would be a retrograde step. The editorial is interesting in its mix of methodological critique of targets with a pragmatic defence of keeping mental health and suicide on a national agenda through the setting of targets. It is also interesting that the critique only extends as far as calling for more clear systems of target setting rather than exploring other ways of interrogating suicide. This methodological mindset has largely dictated how national strategies and policies have been derived since the beginning of the 1990s to the present.

Such uniformity of approach is reflected in the relative lack of variation between countries in the content of suicide prevention strategies (Taylor *et al.*, 1997). An example is the development of different prevention strategies in the four nations of the UK, with England and Scotland adopting strategies in 2002, Northern Ireland in 2006 and Wales in 2008. Despite the possible variance in national contexts these strategies are arguably more marked by their commonality than their diversity. In both form and content, the ways in which policy makers and prevention advisors are presenting approaches to reducing suicide are fairly uniform. We will examine in more detail the English strategy, as an example, but it is worth noting that target groups and explanations of suicidal 'risks' do not vary much between these strategies. What is important for us is how significant factors in suicides have been derived and to ask whether the employment of different methodologies might shed a different light on the most effective ways of combating suicide being seen as a 'reasonable' option for some people.

In order to contextualise our approach and the contribution that it might possibly make to ongoing debates about effective suicide prevention strategies it is worth looking in a little more detail at two examples of work that are currently used by both policy makers and health professionals in England. The relatively uncomplicated 'factual' accounts of antecedents to suicides in key prevention policy documents will then be counterpoised with the more sociological and situated accounts derived from our sociological autopsy study.

Some key documents in English prevention policy

The *National Suicide Prevention Strategy for England* (Department of Health, 2002) is organised around the identification of goals that are targeted to reduce overall rates of suicide. These are: reducing risk in high risk groups; promoting well-being in the wider population; reducing the availability and lethality of suicide methods; improving the reporting of suicide behaviour in the media; promoting research on suicide and suicide prevention and finally the achievement of an overall reduction in numbers of suicides outlined in a government White Paper *Saving Lives: Our Healthier Nation* (Department of Health, 1999). It was this White Paper that drew a strong association between a governmental commitment to improving overall standards of mental well-being and the anticipated concomitant fall in numbers of suicides.

The strategy then moves on to specify the groups and features of suicide that are statistically shown to be of particular concern. The high risk groups are people in contact with mental health services, people who have deliberately self-harmed within the previous year, young men, prisoners and those people in high risk occupational groups – namely farmers, nurses and doctors. Populations targeted for improving well-being include socially excluded and deprived groups, black and ethnic minority groups, people that misuse drugs and/or alcohol, victims and survivors of abuse, children and young people, women during and after pregnancy, older people and those bereaved through suicide. The strategy identifies the statistically most prevalent methods for committing suicide that are targeted – namely hanging and strangulation, self-poisoning, motor vehicle exhaust gas, suicide and railways, jumping from high places and using firearms. The strategy then outlines work on these goals that was ongoing at the time of publication – 2002 – and the plan of work intended over the next decade to achieve target reductions in numbers of suicides as described originally in *Saving Lives: Our Healthier Nation*. The evidence base used here in relation to suicide risk is entirely quantitative. Whilst a national prevention strategy should quite rightly privilege quantitative research in establishing the epidemiology of suicide, the exclusive reliance on quantification is limiting, as it does not allow for the different kinds of insights that qualitative research can bring. In particular, concentrations of risk in particular populations or the prevalence of particular methods can be better *understood* through qualitative inquiry.

In the foreword to the 2008 *National Suicide Prevention Strategy Annual Update* the National Director for Mental Health of the National Mental Health Development Unit, Louis Appleby, asserted that despite an overall fall in numbers of suicides in the general population – including those groups that were identified as high risk in the original strategy – there is no room for complacency. He went on to note that 'periods of high unemployment or severe economic problems have had an adverse effect on the mental health of the population and have been associated with higher rates of suicide' (National Mental Health Development Unit, 2009: 2; see also Gunnell *et al.*, 2009). The association of both socio-economic and pathological antecedents with suicide is clear. However, the social explanations are often subsumed by the pathological. Platt (2011) notes that socio-economic factors are not usually prioritised in prevention strategies, despite strong evidence of the association between socio-economic deprivation and higher suicide rates. This is not to suggest that there is not a relationship between suicide and individual pathology or that mental illness is unimportant. There is a need, however, for a more nuanced approach to the social factors that contribute to people feeling as though they wish to die.

The second document we review here focuses specifically on deaths of people with diagnosed mental illness. *Avoidable Deaths: Five year report of the national confidential inquiry into suicide and homicide by people with mental illness* (National Confidential Inquiry, 2006) is widely used by health professionals such as psychiatrists, NHS managers and psychologists. The intention of the study is to gather information on 'activities of services' and 'patterns of events' prior to suicides and homicides. The Inquiry uses a three stage method. Stage one involves the collection of 'a comprehensive national sample, irrespective of mental health history', the second stage involves the identification of those in the sample that have had contact with mental health services and the third stage involves collection of clinical data about these individuals. For the suicide data, once the deceased have been identified as having had contact with mental health services in the 12 months prior to their death they become 'an inquiry case' and the consultant psychiatrist that dealt with the case is contacted for clinical details. These data are gathered in the form of a 'suicide questionnaire'. The categories on the questionnaire cover: the identification of priority groups; demographic details; clinical history; details of the suicide; details of care in in-patient suicides; details of care in community suicides; details of final contact with patients; respondents' views on prevention; plus there is also space for the psychiatrists to add any additional information (Psychiatry Research Group, University of Manchester, 2010). The point of the report is to ascertain a general picture of rates and methods of suicide of people in contact with mental health services and provide recommendations based on these findings. They found that 27 per cent of all suicides in England and Wales were 'current' or 'recent' mental health patients. Sixty-five per cent of those deaths were caused by hanging/strangulation and self-poisoning – they note that these methods are not falling over time unlike deaths by car exhaust asphyxiation and paracetamol poisoning. The report also collected data on contact with services:

> Forty nine percent of the patients who died had been in contact with services in the previous week, 19% in the previous 24 hours. At the final contact, immediate suicide risk was estimated to be low or absent in 86% of cases.
>
> (National Confidential Inquiry into Suicide and Homicide by People with Mental Illness, 2006: 4)

The report documents a number of falls in rates of deaths in particular circumstances; deaths by strangulation on wards and number of deaths from self-poisoning with tricyclic anti-depressants for example. There are also a number of recommendations made concerning specific mechanisms of mental healthcare practice.

Interesting features of both of these documents – the English suicide prevention strategy and the Confidential Inquiry – are, firstly, the lack of engagement with people from outside the psychiatric health professions and, secondly, the exclusive reliance on statistical data. The whole of this book is concerned with the sociology of suicide so inevitably we will argue for better appreciation of the social context, as a balance to insights from psychiatry and psychology. Much of the rest of the chapter will discuss possible avenues for prevention that arise from our sociological study.

To specifically address the methodological issue at this point, however, it does not appear for instance that any qualitative data have been considered or that wider consultation on methodology took place before the empirical base for these documents was established. The often rehearsed arguments about quantitative versus qualitative methods are well-known, but the idea that they can garner different results is pertinent here. Hjelmeland and Knizek helpfully outline the relationship between 'explanation' and 'understanding' (2010: 75):

> The concepts of *explanations* and *understanding* are interrelated in that causal explanations build on understanding and interpretation, and, to give a causal explanation might be the first step toward developing an understanding. Our point is that these two approaches must be understood on their own terms as interdependent.

To an extent this is the contemporary incarnation of the engagement of Durkheim (suicide as an individual act that could be translated into a social fact through macro-level analysis) and Douglas (the reintroduction of an agent-centred approach to meaning and symbolism in suicide). As we argued in Chapters 2 and 3, we regard sociological dichotomies, such as the opposition of objectivism and subjectivism, social structure and human agency, and the collective and the individual, to be generally unhelpful, and we assert the value of a qualitatively-driven mixed method and dual paradigm approach to the study of suicide. Like Hjelmeland and Knizek we regard explanation and understanding as interdependent. What is striking is that the prevention policy documents reviewed above have eschewed any engagement with the understanding that could be gained via qualitative and mixed methods research.

Our study has suggested particular features of suicides in our cohort which may have been missed without qualitative observations and sociological theorising and which might usefully inform attempts to prevent suicide. At this point we move on to summarise some of these.

Examples from the sociological autopsy study that might inform evolving policy and practice

The insights generated from our qualitatively-driven sociological research might be helpful for policy and practice in several ways. The contribution of studies that seek to understand suicidal events as much as they seek to explain can, in our view, only benefit a deeper engagement with the complex nature of suicide. This is particularly important given that the chances that professionals have for adequately assessing serious suicidal risk appear to be less frequent than might be imagined. As Booth and Owens (2000) observe, studies suggest that anywhere between 65 per cent and 86 per cent of people that kill themselves are not in contact with mental health services when they die. Furthermore, an emphasis on social context is extremely important in preventing suicide. Although undoubtedly mental illness is very often present in suicidal people (Cavanagh *et al.*, 2003), it may well be life events and the social context which trigger suicidal acts, as we have illustrated in Chapters 6 and 7 of this book in particular. Although in the field of suicidology it is fairly mainstream to mention the importance of a bio-psycho-social approach (e.g. Botsis, Soldatos and Costas, 1997), this sometimes seems to be largely lip-service, given that most research is in fact conducted in single disciplines and the 'bio' and the 'psycho' are dominant in the practice of so much research and intervention. In what follows we present some examples of social factors which are highlighted in our research and which warrant attention in preventing suicide.

Relationships with partners

The importance of social relationships, and especially intimate relationships, has emerged as a key theme in our study. Indeed this is a theme that is highlighted in other research (see Stack, 2000b), yet there is no reference to affective relationships in the National Suicide Prevention Strategy for England or a sense that relationships are an appropriate area for policy or strategic intervention. The importance of relationships with significant others, acknowledged by Schneidman (1994b), cannot be underestimated. Whilst it might seem obvious to say, in our study references to partners abound in suicide notes and witness testimony (see Chapters 4 and 5). However, the relational parts of suicide are often subsumed in the language of pathology and individualised accounts which are focused exclusively on the mental health of the deceased. In our study there was some kind of evidence of difficulties or breakdown in relationships with a partner in over half of the cases (see Chapters 3 and 7). The interaction between intimates, and crucially the ways in which these interactions are perceived and acted upon, are important to understanding why a particular repertoire of action might emerge. Attachment theory helps us to conceptualise the central importance of the perception of intimate relationships and responses to their fracture.

All this might suggest that a range of evidence-based interventions focused on intimate relationships might in fact help to prevent suicide. The appropriate intervention would depend on the circumstances. There will be some circumstances where relationship counselling will be suitable, or mediation. Other circumstances where there is domestic abuse might call for more interventions with a clear perpetrator or victim focus. There will be cases where relationship breakdown needs to be managed and others where vulnerable relationships could be maintained with help.

Relationships with children

An interesting finding in our study was the role that children might play in an orientation to suicide. We found that there was often only passing reference to children in accounts of suicides. There was more likely to be a concentration on the trauma caused by splitting up with a partner. This is understandable particularly if it appeared as though the concentration of emotional effort on the part of the person that eventually died is on the breakdown of a relationship. It was interesting then to notice that many suicide notes mentioned children or were specifically addressed to them (see Chapter 5). There were cases where explicit references were made to separation from children and witnesses cited this separation as a reason for the suicide. There were cases where custody battles seemed to loom large, and also those with disputes over financial support for children and contact time. It was also noticeable that even when children were referred to in witness statements, these parts of the testimony were often not dwelt on by those summarising cases. It seemed as though it was not (professional) common sense that the parent-child relationship would loom large amongst possible reasons for suicide.

For us, the simple explanation of single causal factors does not help further understanding of suicidal events. The factoring out of the possible influence of separation from children as a contributory factor in a suicide could potentially be a significant oversight. Whilst adult relationship breakdown may be posited as a causal factor in some studies it may be that a more important source of distress from the split is separation from children that both parties love. In this scenario, the difficult separation is then from people that you want to be with, the children, rather than someone you do not wish to be with, the partner. This issue requires further, more focused, attention in future studies of suicide.

In terms of policies and strategies, we would suggest a much deeper engagement with the meaning of 'family', being a mother, being a father and broader affective relationships. Whilst it is obvious that these are contentious issues, it does not mean that we should not engage with them. People that come into contact with those that are suffering distress – GPs, mental health workers, voluntary sector organisations – would do well to interrogate the aspects of people's lives that may support a particular set of repertoires of action, rather than concentrating on the actor in isolation. Concentrating on how separation or relationships with children contribute to a set of circumstances might prove to be important.

Suicide and the life-course

Problems relating to partners and children were especially concentrated in mid-life, but there were some different issues for the youngest and oldest suicides in our sample. It would seem that young people's suicide threats or attempts might be linked to risk of actual suicide, as might problems in childhood. We suggested a possible connection between a crisis experienced by a young person and problems of attachment. This interpretation would have wider implications for child and family welfare services, such as family support and child protection teams, where the issue of suicide risk is becoming increasingly recognised following the inclusion of youth suicides in serious case reviews (Brandon *et al.*, 2009) and where attachment theory is already widely referenced, even if it is not understood in any depth. For older people in our sample there was an association of suicide with physical illness and bereavement. This might again suggest the need for mainstream services, such as in the fields of primary health care and adult social care, to be alert to suicide risk in physically frail older people, especially in the context of bereavement. It would suggest that the possibility of counselling should be on practitioners' agenda – a need which can easily be overlooked when practical issues and physical care are to the fore in relation to older people's care needs.

Relationship to institutions – health services

There are two very obvious issues with current strategies for suicide prevention that are directly to do with individuals' relationships with health services. One is highlighted by Booth and Owens (2000) where they note the significant proportion of those killing themselves that are not in touch with services at the time of their deaths – prompting the question of why are these people dying and how can interventions be made with people not known to health services? In answer to this question, Booth and Owens suggest two strategies. The first is the use of population-based interventions. The second is a concentration on 'socio-economic deprivation, unemployment and social exclusion' which should lead to a reduction of rates of suicide and self-harm (p. 30). If Booth and Owens are correct, then mental health promotion needs to engage more explicitly with the socio-structural features that support suicidal ideation (see also Platt, 2011).

The second issue to do with individuals' relationship with health services is that of people who kill themselves whilst receiving some limited form of treatment, such as an apparently exclusive use of pharmacological interventions. Socially-rooted distress does not sit easily with the treatment of individualised pathologies. Our qualitative analysis reveals numerous instances where the sorts of social situations people found themselves in could be seen to warrant a degree of unhappiness. However, when it came to medical accounts of the circumstances for suicide these were often simply described as cases of depression or other mental illness. There were cases where, as far as could be told from the inquest evidence, the only treatment had been the prescription of medication (typically SSRIs), despite objectively challenging social circumstances. Although inquest evidence is limited and we cannot be sure there was not a more complex response from health professionals and we have to acknowledge that the deceased themselves may have wanted an exclusively biomedical outcome to their consultation, there is at least an implication here of little or no interrogation of the social context of, say, depression or problem drinking. Health service professionals, in their reports about the deceased, tended to concentrate on narrowly-defined medical antecedents rather than some combination of the medical and the social.

In terms of policy and practice, it important that health services recognise that they are part of a nexus of circumstances that people find themselves in and as such health professionals could be more reflexive about the role they play in suicide. It appears that a reliance on a diagnosis, particularly of depression, often followed by prescription of SSRIs, is not enough in some cases to assist a person through the orientation to suicide to somewhere less dangerous. The consideration of the range of circumstances and experiences that are contributing to an affective state being described as depressed appear as important in some cases as the diagnosis. We would suggest that any diagnosis should ideally be accompanied by a full account of the social circumstances surrounding the individual.

Relationship with institutions – the criminal justice system

Many of the cases that we examined involved various aspects of people's lives being touched by the criminal justice system, including the police and the courts. In 21 per cent of cases the deceased had committed criminal acts and the offending often featured strongly in witness accounts of the context of the suicidal act. There were examples of men who had been charged with possessing child pornography or child sexual abuse and seemed to kill themselves rather than live with the shame of these offences being known. It should be noted in this regard that Pritchard and King's (2004) study of over 1000 coroners' files found that suicide rates in perpetrators of intra- and extra-familial sexual abuse, were 25 and 78 times the general population suicide rate, respectively. The English National Suicide Prevention Strategy notes prisoners and young offenders as key high risk groups. It is well-known that prisoners are vulnerable to suicide. Perhaps what is needed is a rather broader notion of suicide risk in offenders of all ages and at all stages of the criminal justice system, as particularly with stigmatised offences such as child sexual abuse, the act of being arrested or charged can trigger suicide. Suicide risk in offenders raises the general issue that a crude victim-perpetrator dualism can be unhelpful. It may well be that a particular crime has a clear victim and perpetrator, but the offender may well be extremely socially and psychologically vulnerable and as much or more at risk of emotional harm than the victim of the crime. Those working with offenders, such as probation officers, do not need to be told this, but it is more of an issue for general public awareness. That need for greater awareness may include health and social care professionals who occasionally encounter the perpetrator of a crime in routine practice.

Gendered identities and gendered practices

It has already been noted that whilst gender has been identified as an area of concern within suicidology, there has been little or no engagement with the full range of sociological theorising of gender within this field (Scourfield, 2005). Gender tends to be dealt with in an unproblematic way in suicidology. Some facets of gendered behaviour are taken for granted and others ignored. In our qualitatively-driven research we have argued (for example in Chapters 3 and 7) that an understanding of aetiology needs to encompass a range of gendered identities and gendered practices. Prevention strategies should take gender more seriously and engage with the complexity of gender relations in more depth. There is often mention in national prevention strategy documents of particular patterns of suicidal behaviour, e.g. higher rates in men and rising rates (in the late twentieth century) in young men. In practice, service providers tend to be limited in their understanding of gender issues in suicide. There is more to the connections between masculinities and suicide than men's reluctance to ask for help when in distress, for example. The complex array of men's responses to relationship breakdown and work-related problems, for example, are highly relevant.

Holistic responses

Throughout this book we have argued the virtues of a case-based approach to suicide research, which uses rich individual-level data and appreciates the importance of complex individual histories. Chapter 6 in particular emphasises that single-factor explanations are likely to be inadequate and that distress can build up in relation to a series of challenging social circumstances which expand repertoires of action to include the extreme option of suicide. This attention to the whole range of difficulties a person is experiencing supports a holistic view of prevention and treatment. What is needed is work on all aspects of the problem. In all likelihood, few would disagree with this general principle. In practice there are areas in need of improvement, however, such as the over-emphasis on pharmacology and under-playing of social intervention, and the lack of attention to socio-economic factors in national prevention strategies (Platt, 2011).

A holistic approach calls for, amongst other things, working across professional and organisational boundaries. It means collaboration between different groups of professionals with different orientations to service users and work both inside health services and beyond, as argued by Anderson and Jenkins (2006) when discussing the role of nurses in preventing suicide. It calls for a holistic approach to the health care of suicidal individuals which draws on a bio-psycho-social model for understanding mental health and illness (Engel, 1977). Social work, with its eclectic knowledge base, would claim to be the original holistic profession working with people in need. However, the breadth of social work's approach is no longer unique and there has been much work done within health professions to broaden understandings of the causes of ill health. Arguably, then, the basis already exists for the development of more holistic concep-tualisations of individual cases, more inter-professional work and more holistic public health approaches to preventing suicide in communities. There is a need for these approaches to develop, how-ever, and more evidence is needed about the effectiveness of holistic interventions with suicidal people and the effectiveness of multi-factorial public health prevention strategies.

Whilst many health professionals will be familiar with injunc-tions to be less narrowly medical, perhaps more of a challenge for policy and practice is the dual paradigm approach we have argued for. How does a constructionist framing of suicide help with the practical business of preventing suicide? Whilst the practical impli-cations of objectivist research on the aetiology of suicide are more obvious, it would be wrong to conclude that a constructionist approach to suicide has nothing useful to say to practitioners. There are two relevant ideas here. The first is that the practical implica-tions of constructionism have been applied to work with people in need by Parton and O'Byrne (2000), who write about 'constructive social work'. They argue that constructionism implies taking service users' own understandings of their situations very seriously and working closely with these. They recommend therapeutic approaches which engage with how service users see their own situation, such as narrative therapy, helping people to learn to tell different stories about themselves which are oriented to more positive outcomes. The second application of constructionism we recommend is that popular understandings of suicide causation need to be taken seriously. They may be unscientific, but as we have argued at various points through-out the book, the stock of knowledge that inquest witnesses have about why someone might want to kill themselves is likely to be the same stock of knowledge that suicidal people draw upon in deciding how to deal with their distress. Therefore community-level prevention strategies need to engage with the cultural context of suicide and popular understandings of causation and motivations. This could include some careful work with the media and training programmes which aim to increase lay referral of at-risk people for appropriate help. Both of these interventions would benefit from taking lay understandings of suicide causation as one of their starting points.

It should be acknowledged that the arguments above about the need for a holistic approach could be seen, with some justification, as warm words which are much more easily written than they are operationalised. It is, however, beyond the scope of this book to expand in detail on practical approaches to prevention. A multi-professional endeavour is needed to take forward a holistic prevention agenda and this is also beyond the limits of our expertise.

Conclusions

Broadly speaking, three main lessons for prevention emerge from the sociological autopsy study. Firstly, national suicide prevention strategies should consider a broader methodological basis. Strategies can be informed by qualitative research in addition to quantitative epidemiological evidence, to further understanding of suicide and its social contexts. Policy makers report that they value qualitative research (Petticrew *et al.*, 2008) and it is quite possible for qualitative research to be systematically reviewed to reassure sceptics about scale, sampling, validity and reliability (see Popay, Rogers and Williams, 1998; Dixon-Woods and Fitzpatrick, 2001; Thomas *et al.*, 2004).

Secondly, social interventions are needed, to complement medical and psychological treatment. Our study suggests renewed attention should be paid to the breakdown of intimate relationships and adult attachments; parents' loss of children; particular combinations of difficult circumstances at different stages of the life-course; the vulnerability of offenders (and perhaps especially sex offenders) at all stages of the criminal justice process; the large number of suicidal people who have no contact with health services and who might benefit primarily from population-based prevention which is focused on the socio-economic risks; the need for more rounded treatment plans for people with mental health problems which consider social context as well as the need for medication; and the complexity of the whole range of gendered identities and gendered behaviour.

Thirdly, a sociological autopsy approach argues for holistic suicide prevention. This includes bio-psycho-social interventions with suicidal people and inter-disciplinary efforts at community-level prevention. It also includes consideration of how constructionist approaches might inform policy and practice, especially with regard to popular understandings of suicide aetiology – what we might term the *cultural* context of suicide.

References

Adam, K.S. (1973) 'Childhood, parental loss, suicidal ideation and suicidal behavior', in Anthony, E.J. and Koupernik, C. (eds) *The Child in His Family: The Impact of Disease and Death*. New York: Wiley.

Agerbo, E., Stack, S. and Petersen, L. (2009) 'Social integration and suicide trends in Denmark, 1906–2006'. Paper delivered to the annual conference of the American Association of Suicidology, San Francisco, CA., April.

Aggarwal, N. (2008) 'Editorial: Farmer suicides in India: The role of psychiatry and anthropology'. *International Journal of Social Psychiatry*, 54: 291–3.

Ainsworth, M.D.S. (1967) *Infancy in Uganda: Infant Care and the Growth of Love*. Baltimore: John Hopkins University Press.

Ainsworth, M.D.S. (1991) 'Attachment and other affectional bonds across the life cycle', in Parkes, C.M., Stevenson-Hinde, J. and Marris, P. (eds) *Attachment Across the Life Cycle*. New York: Routledge.

Ainsworth, M.D.S., Blehar, M.C., Waters, E. and Wall, S. (1978) *Patterns of Attachment: A Psychological Study of the Strange Situation*. Hillside, NJ: Elbraum.

Allen, R. (2005) 'Statistics on deaths reported to coroners 2004'. *Home Office Statistical Bulletin 2005*. London: Department of Constitutional Affairs.

Anderson, M. and Jenkins, R. (2006) 'The national suicide prevention strategy for England: The reality of a national strategy for the nursing profession'. *Journal of Psychiatric and Mental Health Nursing*, 13(6): 641–50.

Atkinson, J.M. (1978) *Discovering Suicide: Studies in the Social Organization of Sudden Death*. Pittsburgh, PA: University of Pittsburgh Press.

Barraclough, B. and Harris, C. (2002). 'Suicide preceded by murder: The epidemiology of homicide-suicide in England and Wales, 1988–92'. *Psychological Medicine*, 32: 577–84.

Bartholomew, K. (1990) 'Avoidance of intimacy: An attachment perspective'. *Journal of Social and Personal Relationships*, 7: 147–78.

Baudelot, C. and Establet, R. (2008) *Suicide: The Hidden Side of Modernity*. Polity: Cambridge, MA.

Beck, U. and Beck-Gernsheim, E. (1995) *The Normal Chaos of Love*. Cambridge: Polity.

Bell, C. and Newby, H. (1977) *Doing Sociological Research*. London: Allen and Unwin.

Bell, C. and Roberts, H. (1984) *Social Researching*. London: Routledge and Kegan Paul.

Berg, M. and Bowker, G. (1997) 'The multiple bodies of the medical record: Towards a sociology of an artifact'. *Sociological Quarterly*, 38: 513–25.

Berger, P. ([1967] 1990) *The Sacred Canopy: Elements of a Sociological Theory of Religion*. New York: Anchor Books.

Berkman, L.F., Glass, T., Brissette, I. and Seeman, T.E. (2000) 'From social integration to health: Durkheim in the new millennium'. *Social Science and Medicine*, 51(6): 843–57.

Bhaskar, R. ([1979] 1998) *The Possibility of Naturalism: A Philosophical Critique of the Contemporary Human Sciences*. London: Routledge.

Biddle, L. (2003) 'Public hazards or private tragedies? An exploratory study of the effect of coroners' procedures on those bereaved by suicide'. *Social Science and Medicine*, 56: 1033–45.

Biddle, L., Brock, A., Brookes, S.T. and Gunnell, D. (2008) 'Suicide rates in young men in England and Wales in the 21st century: Time trend study'. *British Medical Journal*, 336: 539–42.

Black, S.T. (1993) 'Comparing genuine and simulated notes: A new perspective'. *Journal of Consulting and Clinical Psychology*, 4: 699–702.

Blanchflower, D.G. and Oswald, A.J. (2008) 'Is well-being U-shaped over the life cycle?'. *Social Science and Medicine*, 66: 1733–49.

Bloch, M. and Parry, J.P. (1982) *Death and the Regeneration of Life*. Cambridge: Cambridge University Press.

Blondel, C. (1933) *Le Suicide*. Strassbourg: Librarie Universitaire d'Alsace.

Blumer, H. (1956) 'Sociological analysis and the "variable"'. *American Sociological Review*, 21: 683–90.

Blumer, H. (1969) *Symbolic Interactionism: Perspectives and Method*. Englewood Cliffs: Prentice Hall.

Bocock, R. (2002) *Sigmund Freud*. London: Routledge.

Booth, N. and Owens, C. (2000) 'Silent suicide: Suicide among people not in contact with mental health services'. *International Review of Psychiatry*, 12: 27–30.

Bostik, B.E. and Everall, R.D. (2007) 'Healing from suicide: Adolescent perceptions of attachment relationships'. *British Journal of Guidance and Counselling*, 35(1): 79–96.

Botsis, A.J., Soldatos, C.R. and Costas, S.N. (eds) (1997) *Suicide: Biopsychosocial Approaches*. Amsterdam: Elsevier.

Bourdieu, P. (1980) *Questions de Sociologie*. Paris: Editions de Minuit.

Bourdieu, P. (2001) *Masculine Domination*. Cambridge: Polity.

Bourdieu, P. and de Saint Martin, M. (1982) 'La Sainte Famille. L'episcopat Francais dans le Champ du Puvoir'. *Actes de la Recherché en Sciences Socials*, 44/55: 2–53.

Bourdieu, P. and Wacquant, L.J.D. (1992) *An Invitation to Reflexive Sociology*. Cambridge/Oxford: Polity Press.

Bowlby, J. (1969/1982) *Attachment and Loss, Volume 1: Attachment*. London: Hogarth Press.

Bowlby, J. (1973) *Attachment and Loss, Volume 2: Separation: Anxiety and Anger*. London: Hogarth Press.

Bradbury, M. (1996) 'Representations of "good" and "bad" deaths among death-workers and the bereaved', in Howarth, G. and Jupp, P.C. (eds) *Contemporary Issues in the Sociology of Death, Dying and Disposal*. Basingstoke: Macmillan.

Brandon, M., Bailey, S., Belderson, P., Gardner, R., Sidebotham, P., Dodsworth, J., Warren, J. and Black, J. (2009) *Understanding Serious Case Reviews and Their*

Impact: A Biennial Analysis of Serious Case Reviews 2005–7, Research report DCSF-RR129. London: DCFS.

Breault, K.D. (1994) 'Was Durkheim right? A critical survey of the empirical literature on le suicide', in Lester, D. (ed.) *Emile Durkheim, Le Suicide: 100 Years Later*. Philadelphia: The Charles Press.

Bryman, A. (1988) *Quantity and Quality in Social Research*. London: Routledge.

Bryman, A. (2004) *Social Research Methods*. Oxford: Oxford University Press.

Burawoy, M. (2005) '2004 Presidential address: For public sociology'. *American Sociological Review*, 70(1): 4–28.

Canetto, S.S. (1995) 'Men who survive a suicidal act: Successful coping or failed masculinity?', in Sabo, D. and Gordon, D. (eds) *Men's Health and Illness: Gender, Power, and the Body*, pp. 292–304. Newbury Park, CA: Sage.

Canetto, S.S. (1992–3) 'She died for love and he for glory: Gender myths of suicidal behavior'. *Omega: The Journal of Death and Dying*, 26(1): 1–17.

Canetto, S.S. (1997) 'Gender and suicidal behavior: Theories and evidence', in Maris, R.W., Silverman, M.M. and Canetto, S.S. (eds) *Review of Suicidology*, pp. 138–67. New York: Guilford.

Canetto, S.S. and Lester, D. (2002) 'Love and achievement motives in women's and men's suicide notes'. *Journal of Psychology*, 136: 573–6.

Cantor, C. (2000) 'Suicide in the western world', in Hawton, K. and van Heeringen, K. (eds) *The International Handbook of Suicide and Attempted Suicide*, pp. 9–28. London: Wiley.

Carmin, J. and Balser, D. (2002) 'Selecting repertoires of action in social movement organizations'. *Organization and Environment*, 15(4): 365–88.

Cassidy, J. and Shaver, P.R. (2008) *Handbook of Attachment: Theory, Research and Clinical Applications*. New York: The Guilford Press.

Cattell, H. (2000) 'Suicide in the elderly'. *Advances in Psychiatric Treatment*, 6: 102–8.

Cavan, R.S. (1965 [1928]) *Suicide*. New York: Russell and Russell.

Cavanagh, J.T., Carson, A.J., Sharpe, M. and Lawrie, S.M. (2003) 'Psychological autopsy studies of suicide: A systematic review'. *Psychological Medicine*, 33(3): 395–405.

Chatterjee, P. and Bailey, D. (1993) 'False empowerment: Lessons from three sociological autopsies of community action'. *Case Analysis*, 3(2): 113–31.

Coleman, J.C. and Hendry, L. (1999) *The Nature of Adolescence*. London: Routledge.

Connell, R.W. (1995) *Masculinities*. Cambridge: Polity.

Connell, R.W. (2002) 'On hegemonic masculinity and violence: A response to Jefferson and Hall'. *Theoretical Criminology*, 6(1): 89–99.

Coyle, A. and Morgan-Sykes, C. (1998) 'Troubled men and threatening women: The construction of crisis in male mental health'. *Feminism and Psychology*, 8(3).

Coyle, J. and MacWhannell, D. (2002) 'The importance of "morality" in the social construction of suicide in Scottish newspapers'. *Sociology of Health and Illness*, 24(6): 689–713.

Crowell, J.A., Fraley, R.C. and Shaver, P.R. (2008) 'Measurement of individual differences in adolescent and adult attachment', in Cassidy, J. and Shaver, P.R.

(2008) *Handbook of Attachment: Theory, Research and Clinical Applications.* New York: The Guilford Press.

Davis, G., Lindsay, R., Seabourne, G. and Griffiths-Baker, J. (2002) 'Experiencing inquests'. *Home Office Research Study 241.* London: Home Office Research, Development and Statistics Directorate.

de Jong, M.L. (1992) 'Attachment, individuation and risk of suicide in late adolescence'. *Journal of Youth and Adolescence*, 21(3): 357–73.

Department of Health (1999) *Saving Lives: Our Healthier Nation.* London: HMSO.

Department of Health (2002) *The National Suicide Prevention Strategy for England.* London: Department of Health.

Dixon-Woods, M. and Fitzpatrick, R. (2001) 'Qualitative research in systematic reviews has established a place for itself'. *British Medical Journal*, 323: 765–6.

Dobash, R.E. and Dobash, R.P. (1979) *Violence Against Wives.* New York: Free Press.

Dorries, C.P. (2004) *Coroners' Courts: A Guide to Law and Practice.* Oxford, New York: Oxford University Press.

Douglas, J. (1967) *The Social Meanings of Suicide.* Princeton: Princeton University Press.

Dozier, M., Stovall-McClough, K.C. and Albus, K.E. (2008) 'Attachment and psychopathology', in Cassidy, J. and Shaver, P.R. (2008) *Handbook of Attachment: Theory, Research and Clinical Applications.* New York: The Guilford Press.

Dumit, J. (1997) 'A digital image of the person', in Downey, G.L. and Dumit, J. (eds) *Cyborgs and Citadels: Anthropological Interventions in Emerging Sciences and Technologies.* Santa Fe, N.M.: School of American Research.

Duneier, M. (2006) 'Ethnography, the ecological fallacy, and the 1995 Chicago Heat Wave'. *American Sociological Review*, 71: 679–88.

Durkheim, E. (2002 [1897]) *Suicide: A Study in Sociology.* London: Routledge.

Engel, G.L. (1977) 'The need for a new medical model: A challenge for biomedicine'. *Science*, 196(4286): 129–36.

Feeney, B.C. and Monin, J.K. (2008) 'An attachment-theoretical perspective on divorce', in Cassidy, J. and Shaver, P.R. (2008) *Handbook of Attachment: Theory, Research and Clinical Applications.* New York: The Guilford Press.

Fincham, B., Scourfield, J. and Langer, S. (2007) 'Documentary data: Single medium, multiple modes?'. *Qualitative Researcher*, 5: 2–4.

Fincham, B., Scourfield, J. and Langer, S. (2008) 'The impact of working with disturbing secondary data: Reading suicide files in a coroner's office'. *Qualitative Health Research*, 18: 853–62.

Fine, G.A. (1997) 'Scandal, social conditions and the creation of public attention: Fatty Arbuckle and the "Problem of Hollywood"'. *Social Problems*, 44(3): 297–323.

Fine, G.A. (2007) 'The construction of historical equivalence: Weighing the Red and Brown Scares'. *Symbolic Interaction*, 30(1): 27–39.

Fonagy, P., Gergely, G. and Target, M. (2008) 'Psychoanalytic constructs and attachment theory and research', in Cassidy, J. and Shaver, P.R. (2008) *Handbook of Attachment: Theory, Research and Clinical Applications.* New York: The Guilford Press.

Foucault, M. (1994 [1973]) *The Birth of the Clinic: An Archaeology of Medical Perception*. New York: Vintage Books.

Fraley, R.C., Brumbaugh, C.C. and Marks, M.J. (2005) 'The evolution and function of adult attachment: A comparative and phylogenetic analysis', *Journal of Personality and Social Psychology*, 89: 731–46.

Freud, S. (1953) 'Thoughts for the times on war and death', in *The Standard Edition of the Complete Psychological Works of Sigmund Freud*, Vol. IV. London: Hogarth Press.

Friedman, S. (1968) 'Suicide'. *Journal of the American Medical Association*, 204(6): 232.

Fullager, S. (2003) 'Wasted lives'. *Journal of Sociology*, 39: 291–307.

Furlong, A. and Cartmel, F. (2007) *Young People and Social Change: New Perspectives*. Maidenhead: Open University Press.

Gavin, M. and Rogers, A. (2006) 'Narratives of suicide in psychological autopsy: Bringing lay knowledge back in'. *Journal of Mental Health*, 15(2): 135–44.

Gell, A. (1998) *Art and Agency: An Anthropological Theory*. Oxford: Clarendon.

Gibbs, J. (1994) 'Durkheim's heavy hand in the sociological study of suicide', in Lester, D. (ed.) *Emile Durkheim, Le Suicide: 100 Years Later*. Philadelphia: The Charles Press.

Giddens, A. (1965) 'The suicide problem in French sociology', *The British Journal of Sociology*, 16(1): 3–18.

Giddens, A. (1971) 'A typology of suicide', in Giddens, A. (ed.) *The Sociology of Suicide: A Selection of Readings*. London: Frank Cass and Co.

Giddens, A. (1976) *New Rules of Sociological Method: A Positive Critique of Interpretative Sociologies*. London: Hutchinson.

Giddens, A. (1984) *The Constitution of Society: Outline of the Theory of Structuration*. Cambridge: Polity Press.

Giddens, A. (1992) *The Transformation of Intimacy*. Cambridge: Polity.

Giddens, A. (2006) *Sociology*. Cambridge: Polity.

Gilbert, N. (2008) *Researching Social Life*. London: Sage.

Gilchrist, E., Johnson, R., Takriti, R., Beech, A., Kebbell, M. and Weston, S. (2003) 'Domestic violence offenders characteristics and offending related needs', Findings No. 217. London: Home Office.

Girdhar, S., Leenaars, A.A., Dogra, T.D., Leenaars, L. and Kumar, G. (2004) 'Suicide notes in India: What do they tell us?'. *Archives of Suicide Research*, 8: 179–85.

Goffman, E. (1959) *The Presentation of Self in Everyday Life*. New York: Doubleday Anchor.

Gold, M. (1958) 'Suicide, homicide and the socialisation of aggression'. *The American Journal of Sociology*, LXII: 651–61.

Gubrium, J. (1993) 'For a cautious naturalism', in Holstein, J.A. and Miller, G. (eds) *Reconsidering Social Constructionism*, pp. 55–68. Hawthorn, NY: Aldine de Gruyter.

Gunnell, D., Middleton, N., Whitley, E., Frankel, S. and Dorling, D. (2003) 'Why are suicide rates in young men increasing but falling in the elderly? A time series analysis of trends in England and Wales 1950–1998'. *Social Science and Medicine*, 57: 595–611.

Gunnell, D., Platt, S. and Hawton, K. (2009) 'The economic crisis and suicide'. *British Medical Journal*, 338: 1456–7.

Gurvitch, G. (1939) *Essais de Sociologie*. Paris: Librarie du Recueil Sirey.

Hallam, E., Hockey, J.L. and Howarth, G. (1999) *Beyond the Body: Death and Social Identity*. London, New York: Routledge.

Hammersley, M. (1992) *What's Wrong With Ethnography*. London: Routledge.

Hammersley, M. (1996) 'The relationship between qualitative and quantitative research: Paradigm loyalty versus methodological eclecticism', in Richardson, J.T.E. (ed.) *Handbook of Research Methods for Psychology and the Social Sciences*. Leicester: BPS Books.

Hammersley, M. and Gomm, R. (1997) 'Bias in social research'. *Sociological Research Online*, 1(2): http://www.socresonline.org.uk/2/1/2.html

Handelman, L.D. and Lester, D. (2007) 'The content of suicide notes from attempters and completers'. *Crisis*, 28(2): 102–4.

Harris, O. (1982) 'The dead and the devils among the Bolivian Laymi', in Bloch, M. and Parry, J.P. (eds) *Death and the Regeneration of Life*. Cambridge: Cambridge University Press.

Hawton, K. (1998) 'A national target for reducing suicide'. *British Medical Journal*, 317: 156–7.

Hawton, K. and van Heeringen, K. (eds) (2000) *The International Handbook of Suicide and Attempted Suicide*. London: Wiley.

Hawton, K., Appleby, L., Platt, S., Foster, T., Cooper, J., Malmberg, A. and Simkin, S. (1998) 'The psychological autopsy approach to studying suicide: A review of methodological issues'. *Journal of Affective Disorders*, 50(2–3): 269–76.

Helliwell, J. (2007) 'Well-being and social capital: Does suicide pose a puzzle?'. *Social Indicators Research*, 81(3): 455–96.

Hendin, H. (1991) 'Psychodynamics of suicide, with particular reference to the young'. *American Journal of Psychiatry*, 148: 1150–8.

Henry, A.F. and Short, J.F. (1954) *Suicide and Homicide: Some Economic, Sociological and Psychological Aspects of Aggression*. Glencoe: The Free Press.

Hertz, R. (1960) *Death and the Right Hand*. Aberdeen: Cohen and West.

Hesse, E. (2008) 'The adult attachment interview: Protocol, method of analysis, and empirical studies', in Cassidy, J. and Shaver, P.R. (2008) *Handbook of Attachment: Theory, Research and Clinical Applications*. New York: The Guilford Press.

Hirshci, T. (1969) *Causes of Delinquency*. Berkeley: University of California Press.

Hjelmeland, H. and Knizek, B.L. (2010) 'Why we need qualitative research in suicidology'. *Suicide and Life-Threatening Behaviour*, 40(1): 74–80.

Hockey, J. and Draper, J. (2005) 'Beyond the womb and the tomb: Identity, (dis)embodiment and the life course'. *Body and Society*, 11: 41–58.

Hockey, J.L., Kellehar, L. and Prendergast, D. (2007) 'Sustaining kinship: Ritualization and the disposal of human ashes in the United Kingdom', in Mitchell, M. (ed.) *Remember Me, Constructing Immortality: Beliefs on Immortality, Life, and Death*. London: Routledge.

Holmes, J. (1993) *John Bowlby and Attachment Theory*. London: Routledge.

Holmes, J. (2001) *The Search for the Secure Base*. London: Routledge.

Howarth, G. (1996) *Last Rites: The Work of The Modern Funeral Director*. Amityville, N.Y.: Baywood Pub. Co.

Howarth, G. (2007) *Death and Dying: A Sociological Introduction*. Cambridge: Polity.

Jacobs, J. (1967) 'A phenomenological study of suicide notes'. *Social Problems*, 15(1): 60–72.

Jenkins, R. (1992) *Pierre Bourdieu*. London: Routledge.

Jenks, C. (1998) *Core Sociological Dichotomies*. London: Sage.

Johnson, K. and Fincham, B. (2008) 'Lost in translation: Communication and suicidal behaviours'. Presentation to the Ethnographies of Suicide Conference at Brunel University, 2nd–3rd July.

Joiner, T.E. (2005) *Why People Die By Suicide?*. Cambridge, MA: Harvard University Press.

Jones, N.J. and Bennell, C. (2007) 'The development and validation of statistical prediction rules for discriminating between genuine and simulated suicide notes'. *Archives of Suicide Research*, 11: 219–33.

Joralemon, D. (1995) 'Organ wars: The battle for body parts'. *Medical Anthropology Quarterly*, 9: 335–56.

Kirk, J. and Miller, M.L. (1986) *Reliability and Validity in Qualitative Research*. Newbury Park, CA: Sage.

Klinenberg, E. (2002). *Heat Wave: A Social Autopsy of Disaster in Chicago*. Chicago: Chicago University Press.

Klinenberg, E. (2006) 'Blaming the victims: Hearsay, labeling, and the hazards of quick-hit disaster ethnography'. *American Sociological Review*, 71: 689–98.

Knizek, B.L. and Hjelmeland, H. (2007) 'A theoretical model for interpreting suicidal behaviour as communication'. *Theory and Psychology*, 17: 697–720.

Kress, G. and Van Leeuwen, T. (2001) *Multimodal Discourse: The Modes and Media of Contemporary Communication*. London: Arnold.

Kushner, H.I. (1993) 'Suicide, gender, and the fear of modernity in nineteenth-century medical and social thought'. *Journal of Social History*, 26(3): 461–90.

Kushner, H.I. (1994) 'Durkheim and the immunity of women to suicide', in Lester, D. (ed.) *Emile Durkheim, Le Suicide: 100 Years Later*. Philadelphia: The Charles Press.

Langer, S. (2010) 'Distributed personhood and the transformation of agency: An anthropological perspective on inquests', in Hockey, J., Komaromy, C. and Woodthorpe, K. (eds) *The Matter of Death: Space, Place and Materiality*. Basingstoke: Palgrave Macmillan.

Laub, J.H. and Sampson, R.J. (2003) *Shared Beginnings, Divergent Lives: Delinquent Boys to Age 70*. Cambridge, Massachusetts: Harvard University Press.

Law, J. (2004) *After Method: Mess in Social Science Research*. London: Routledge.

Ledgerwood, D.M. (1999) 'Suicide and attachment: Fear of abandonment: and isolation from a developmental perspective'. *Journal of Contemporary Psychotherapy*, 29(1): 65–73.

Leenaars, A.A. (2003) 'Can a theory of suicide predict elderly suicides?'. *Crisis*, 24(1): 7–16.

Leenaars, A.A., Sayin, A., Candansayar, S., Leenaars, L., Akar, T. and Demirel, B. (2010) 'Suicide in different cultures: A thematic comparison of suicide notes from Turkey and the United States'. *Journal of Cross-Cultural Psychology*, 42: 253–63.

Leenaars, A.A. (1988) *Suicide Notes*. New York: Human Sciences Press.

Leenars, A.A., Lester, D., Wenckstern, S., McMullin, C., Rudzinski, D. and Brevard, A. (1992) 'Comparisons of suicide notes and parasuicide notes'. *Death Studies*, 16: 331–41.

Lester, D. (1994) *Emile Durkheim, Le Suicide: One Hundred Years Later*. Philadelphia: Charles Press.

Liebling, A. (1992) *Suicides in Prison*. London: Routledge.

Lindqvist, P. and Gustafsson, L. (2002) 'Suicide classification – clues and their use: A study of 122 cases of suicide and undetermined manner of death'. *Forensic Science International*, 128: 136–40.

Lyon, M.E., Benoit, M., O'Donnell, R.M., Getson, P.R, Siber, T. and Walsh, T. (2000) 'Assessing African American adolescents' risk for suicide attempts: Attachment theory'. *Adolescence*, 35(137): 121–34.

Magai, C. (2008) 'Attachment in middle and later life', in Cassidy, J. and Shaver, P.R. (2008) *Handbook of Attachment: Theory, Research and Clinical Applications*. New York: The Guilford Press.

Maimon, D. and Kuhl, D.C. (2008) 'Social control and youth suicidality: Situating Durkheim's ideas in a multilevel framework'. *American Sociological Review*, 73(6): 921–43.

Maris, R. (1981) *Pathways to Suicide*. Baltimore, MD: John Hopkins University Press.

Mason, J. (2006) 'Mixing methods in a qualitatively-driven way'. *Qualitative Research*, 6(1): 9–25.

McClelland, L., Reicher, S. and Booth, N. (2000) 'A last defence: The negotiation of blame within suicide notes'. *Journal of Community and Applied Social Psychology*, 10: 225–40.

McMahon, A. (1999) *Taking Care of Men: Sexual Politics in the Public Mind*. Cambridge: Cambridge University Press.

Mecke, V. (2004) *Fatal Attachments: The Instigation to Suicide*. Prager: Westport, Conn.

Meloy, J.R. (1998) *The Psychology of Stalking: Clinical and Forensic Perspectives*. New York: Academic Press.

Meltzer, H., Lader, D., Corbin, T., Singleton, N., Jenkins, R. and Brugha, T. (2002) *Non-fatal Suicidal Behaviour among Adults Aged 16 to 74 in Great Britain*. London: Stationery Office.

National Confidential Inquiry in Suicide and Homicide by People with Mental Illness (2006) *Avoidable Deaths: Five Year Report of the National Confidential Inquiry Into Suicide and Homicide By People With Mental Illness*. http://www.medicine.manchester.ac.uk/suicideprevention/nci/Useful/avoidable_deaths.pdf [accessed 22.03.2010].

National Mental Health Development Unit (2009) *National Suicide Prevention Strategy for England: Annual Report on Progress 2008*. Leeds: NMHDU.

O'Carroll, P.W. (1989) 'A consideration of the validity and reliability of suicide mortality data'. *Suicide and Life-Threatening Behaviour*, 19: 1–16.

Oakley, A. (1999) 'Paradigm wars: Some thoughts on a personal and public trajectory'. *International Journal of Social Research Methodology*, 2(3): 247–54.

O'Connor, R. and Leenaars, A.A. (2004) 'A thematic comparison of suicide notes drawn from Northern Ireland and the United States'. *Current Psychology: Developmental, Learning, Personality, Social*, 22(4): 229–347.

O'Donnell, I., Farmer, R. and Catalan, J. (1993) 'Suicide notes'. *British Journal of Psychiatry*, 163: 45–8.

Office for National Statistics (2001) *Mortality Statistics: Cause. Review of the Registrar General on Deaths by Cause, Sex and Age, in England and Wales, 2000*. London: Office for National Statistics.

Office for National Statistics [ONS] (2010a) *Mortality Statistics: Deaths Registered in 2008. Review of the National Statistician on Deaths in England and Wales*. London: Crown Copyright. http://www.statistics.gov.uk/statbase/Product. asp?vlnk=15096 (accessed April 2 2010).

Office for National Statistics [ONS] (2010b) *Divorces in England and Wales 2008*. Newport: Office for National Statistics. http://www.statistics.gov.uk/statbase/ Product.asp?vlnk=14124 (accessed April 2 2010).

Office of National Statistics (2007) 'Use of ICT at home'. *Focus on the Digital Age*. London: HMSO.

Owen, K. (2003) 'Mad, bad or just plain sad dads: The relationship of post-separation parenting patterns and grief on the mental and physical health of fathers', in Sullivan, R. (ed.) *Focus on Fathering*. London: Routledge.

Owens, C., Lambert, H., Lloyd, K. and Donovan, J. (2008) 'Tales of biographical disintegration: How parents make sense of their sons' suicides'. *Sociology of Health and Illness*, 30: 237–54.

Parton, N. and O'Byrne, P. (2000) *Constructive Social Work*. Basingstoke: Palgrave Macmillan.

Payne, G. and Williams, M. (2005) 'Generalization in qualitative research'. *Sociology*, 39: 295–314.

Payne, G., Williams, M. and Chamberlain, S. (2004) 'Methodological pluralism in British sociology'. *Sociology*, 38(1): 153–63.

Pescosolido, B.A. and Mendelsohn, R. (1986) 'Social causation or social construction of suicide? An investigation into the social organization of official rates'. *American Sociological Review*, 51(1): 80–101.

Pescosolido, B.A. (1994) 'Bringing Durkheim into the twenty-first century: A network approach to unresolved issues in the Sociology of Suicide', in Lester, D. (ed.) *Emile Durkheim, Le Suicide: 100 Years Later*. Philadelphia: The Charles Press.

Petticrew, M., Platt, S., McCollam, A., Wilson, S. and Thomas, S. (2008) 'We're not short of people telling us what the problems are. We're short of people telling us what to do: An appraisal of public policy and mental health'. *BMC Public Health*, 8: 314.

Pickering, W.S.F. and Walford, G. (2000) *Durkheim's Suicide: A Century of Research and Debate*. London: Routledge.

Platt, S. (2011) 'Inequalities and suicidal behaviour', in O'Connor, R., Platt, S. and Gordon, J. (eds) *International Handbook of Suicide Prevention: Research, Policy and Practice*. Oxford: Wiley-Blackwell.

Platt, S., Backett, S. and Kreitman, N. (1988) 'Social construction or causal ascription: Distinguishing suicide from undetermined death'. *Social Psychiatry and Psychiatric Epidemiology*, 23: 217–21.

Platt, S. and Hawton, K. (2000) 'Suicidal behaviour and the labour market', in Hawton, K. and van Heeringen, K. (eds) *The International Handbook of Suicide and Attempted Suicide*, pp. 309–84. London: Wiley.

Popay, J., Rogers, A. and Williams, G. (1998) 'Rationale and standards for the systematic review of qualitative literature in health services research'. *Qualitative Health Research*, 8(3): 431–51.

Prior, L. (1985) 'The good, the bad and the unnatural: A study of coroners' decisions in Northern Ireland'. *The Sociological Review*, 33: 64–90.

Prior, L. (1987) 'Policing the dead – a sociology of the mortuary'. *Sociology*, 21: 355–76.

Pritchard, C. and King, E. (2004) 'A comparison of child-sex-abuse-related and mental-disorder-related suicide in a six-year cohort of regional suicides: The importance of the child protection-psychiatric interface'. *British Journal of Social Work*, 34(2): 181–98.

Psychiatry Research Group, University of Manchester (2010) 'Core suicide/Homicide method' http://www.medicine.manchester.ac.uk/psychiatry/research/suicide/prevention/nci/methods [accessed 22.03.2010].

Rapport, N. (2009) 'Ethics of apology', in Mookherjee, N., Rapport, N., Josephides, L., Hage, G., Renier Todd, L. and Cowlinshaw, G. (2009) 'The ethics of apology: A set of commentaries'. *Critique of Anthropology*, 29(3): 345–66.

Redfield, J.K. (2000) *Night Falls Fast: Understanding Suicide*. New York: Vintage.

Redman, P. (2008) *Attachment: Sociology and Social Worlds*. Manchester: Manchester University Press.

Reed, A. (2006) 'Documents unfolding', in Riles, A. (ed.) *Documents: Artifacts of Modern Knowledge*. Ann Arbor: University of Michigan Press.

Reiner, R. (2007) 'Political economy, crime and criminal justice', in Maguire, M., Morgan, R. and Reiner, R. (eds) *The Oxford Handbook of Criminology*. Oxford: Oxford University Press.

Richardson, R. (2000) *Death, Dissection and the Destitute*. Chicago and London: Chicago University Press.

Riles, A. (2001) *The Network Inside Out*. Ann Arbor: University of Michigan Press.

Riles, A. (ed.) (2006a) *Documents: Artifacts of Modern Knowledge*. Ann Arbor: University of Michigan Press.

Riles, A. (2006b) 'Introduction: In response', in Riles, A. (ed.) *Documents: Artifacts of Modern Knowledge*. Ann Arbor: University of Michigan Press.

Robertson, M. (2006) 'Books reconsidered: Emile Durkheim, *Le Suicide*'. *Australasian Psychiatry*, 14(4): 365–8.

Rock, P. (2005) 'Chronocentrism and British criminology'. *The British Journal of Sociology*, 56(3): 473–91.

Rutter, M. (2006) 'Critical notice: Attachment from infancy: The major longitudinal studies'. *Journal of Child Psychology and Psychiatry*, 47: 974–7.

Rutter, M. (2008) 'Implications of attachment theory and research for child care policies', in Cassidy, J. and Shaver, P.R. (2008) *Handbook of Attachment: Theory, Research and Clinical Applications*. New York: The Guilford Press.

Sainsbury, P. and Jenkins, J.S. (1982) 'The accuracy of officially reported suicide statistics for purposes of epidemiological research'. *Journal of Epidemiology and Community Health*, 36: 43–8.

Sainsbury, P. and Barraclough, B.M. (1968) 'Differences between suicide rates'. *Nature*, 220: 1232.

Salib, E., Cawley, S. and Healy, R. (2002) 'The significance of suicide notes in the elderly'. *Aging and Mental Health*, 6(2): 186–90.

Sanger, S. and McCarthy Veach, P. (2008) 'The interpersonal nature of suicide: A qualitative investigation of suicide notes'. *Archives of Suicide Research*, 12: 353–65.

Scheper-Hughes, N. (1992) *Death Without Weeping: The Violence of Everyday Life in Brazil*. Berkeley, Oxford: University of California Press.

Schneidman, E. (1969) 'Suicide, lethality, and the psychological autopsy'. *International Psychiatry Clinics*, 6(2): 225–50.

Schneidman, E. (1994a) 'The psychological autopsy'. *American Psychologist*, 49(1): 75–6.

Schneidman, E. (1994b) *Definition of Suicide*. Northvale: Jason Aronson Inc.

Schneidman, E.S. and Farberow, N.L. (1957) 'Some comparisons between genuine and simulated notes'. *Journal of General Psychology*, 56: 251–6.

Schutz, A. (1953) 'Common-sense and scientific interpretation in human action'. *Philosophy and Phenomenological Research*, 14: 1–38.

Scottish Executive (2002) *Choose Life: A National Strategy and Action Plan to Prevent Suicide in Scotland*. Edinburgh: Scottish Executive.

Scourfield, J. (2005) 'Suicidal masculinities'. *Sociological Research Online*, 10(2), http://www.socresonline.org.uk/10/2/scourfield.html accessed 13.10.2010.

Sibeon, R. (1999) 'Anti-reductionist sociology'. *Sociology*, 33(2): 317–24.

Silverman, A.B., Reinherz, H.Z. and Giaconia, R.M. (1996) 'The long-term sequelae of child and adolescent abuse: A longitudinal community study'. *Child Abuse and Neglect*, 20(8): 709–23.

Silverman, D. (2001) *Interpreting Qualitative Data: Methods for Analysing Talk, Text and Interaction*. London: Sage.

Simpson, G. (1951) 'Editor's introduction: The aetiology of suicide', in Durkheim, E. (1951) *Suicide: A Study in Sociology*. London and New York: The Free Press.

Slater, G.Y. (2005) 'Firearm suicide among older adults: A sociological autopsy'. Unpublished PhD thesis, Indiana University.

Smith, D.J. (1994) 'Race, crime and criminal justice', in Maguire, M., Morgan, R. and Reiner, R. (eds) *The Oxford Handbook of Criminology*. Oxford: Clarendon.

Stack, S. (1994) 'Reformulating Durkheim: 100 years later', in Lester, D. (ed.) *Emile Durkheim, Le Suicide: 100 Years Later*. Philadelphia: The Charles Press.

Stack, S. (2000a) 'Suicide: A 15 year review of the sociological literature: Part I: Cultural and economic factors'. *Suicide and Life Threatening Behavior*, 30(2): 145–62.

Stack, S. (2000b) 'Suicide: A 15 year review of the sociological literature, Part II: Modernization and social integration perspectives'. *Suicide and Life Threatening Behavior*, 30(2): 163–76.

Stack, S. and Wasserman, I. (2007) 'Economic strain and suicide risk: A qualitative analysis'. *Suicide and Life-Threatening Behavior*, 37(1): 103–12.

Stengel, E. (1958) *Attempted Suicide: Its Social Significance and Effects*. London: Chapman and Hall.

Strathern, M. (1992) *After Nature: English Kinship in the Late Twentieth Century*. Cambridge: Cambridge University Press.

Taylor, S. (1994) 'Suicide and social theory', in Lester, D. (ed.) *Emile Durkheim, Le Suicide: 100 Years Later*. Philadelphia: The Charles Press.

Taylor, S.J., Kingdom, D. and Jenkins, R. (1997) 'How are nations trying to prevent suicide? An analysis of national suicide prevention strategies'. *Acta Psychiatrica Scandinavica*, 95: 457–63.

Thomas, J., Harden, A., Oakley, A., Oliver, S., Sutcliffe, K., Rees, R., Brunton, G. and Kavanagh, J. (2004) 'Integrating qualitative research with trials in systematic reviews'. *British Medical Journal*, 328: 1010–12.

Thompson, R.A. (2008) 'Early attachment and later development: Familiar questions, new answers', in Cassidy, J. and Shaver, P.R. (2008) *Handbook of Attachment: Theory, Research and Clinical Applications*. New York: The Guilford Press.

Timmermans, S. (2005) 'Suicide determination and the professional authority of medical examiners'. *American Sociological Review*, 70(2): 311–33.

Utriainen, T. and Honkasalo, M-L. (1996) 'Women writing their death and dying: Semiotic perspectives on women's suicide notes'. *Semiotica*, 109(3/4): 195–220.

Van Orden, K.A., Witte, T.K., Gordon, K.H., Bender, T.W. and Joiner, T.E. (2008) 'Suicidal desire and the capability for suicide: Tests of the interpersonal-psychological theory of suicidal behaviour among adults'. *Journal of Consulting and Clinical Psychology*, 76(1): 72–83.

Violato, C. and Arato, J. (2004) 'Childhood attachment and adolescent suicide: A stepwise discriminant analysis in a case comparison study'. *Individual Differences Research*, 2(3): 162–8.

Wacquant, L. (1992) 'Toward a social praxeology: The structure and logic of Bourdieu's sociology', in Bourdieu, P. and Wacquant, L. (eds) *An Invitation to Reflexive Sociology*. Oxford: Polity Press.

Wainwright, D. and Calnan, M. (2008) *Work Stress: The Making of a Modern Epidemic*. Maidenhead: Open University.

Ward, T. and Maruna, S. (2007) *Rehabilitation*. London: Routledge.

Wertheimer, A. (1990) *A Special Scar: The Experiences of People Bereaved by Suicide*. London: Routledge.

Whitehead, S. (2002) *Men and Masculinities*. Cambridge: Polity

Whitt, H.P. (2006) 'Where did the bodies go? The social construction of suicide data, New York City, 1976–92'. *Sociological Inquiry*, 76(2): 166–87.

Wong, W.C., Yeung, A.W.M. and Chang, W.S.C. (2009) 'Suicide notes in Hong Kong in 2000'. *Death Studies*, 33: 372–81.

Wright Mills, C. (1959) *The Sociological Imagination*. Oxford: Oxford University Press.

Zonda, T. (1999) 'Suicide in Nógrád County, Hungary, 1970–1994'. *Crisis*, 20(2): 64–70.

Index

adolescence, 148, 153
affective dimension, 131
age, suicide by, 145–6, 148
age-graded theory, of informal
      social control, 136
agency–structure interplay, 137
Ainsworth, M.D.S., 138–9
altruistic suicide, 10, 12–13, 29
ambivalence toward parent, 142
anomic suicide, 10, 12–13, 36
anti-reductionist sociology, 47
apologies, 170
   in suicide notes as connection,
      94–100
Atkinson, J.M., 3
   *Discovering Suicide: Studies in the
      Social Organization of Sudden
      Death*, 23–7
attachment theory, 136, 138–44,
      151, 164, 179

bad death, 96
bereavement, 53, 96, 158, 165
bio-psycho-social approach, 178,
      184
blame, 87
Blumer, H., 39–40
Bourdieu, P., 32
Bowlby, J., 138–9, 141
Bryman, A., 41

Cavan, Ruth S.
   Suicide, 15 18
children, separation from, 179–80
childhood experiences, 154
child-parent relationship, 142,
      178–9
clusters of circumstances, and
      suicide, 111
   case studies, 115, 120, 125, 129
collective conscience, 10

collective representations, 35,
      45
common sense theories, 20, 25,
      55–8
community organisation, and
      suicide, 16
consciousness, individual, 34
constructionism, 43, 184
Coroners Rules, 69, 71
coroners' files, 174
   making sense of, 52–4
   see also reports
criminal justice system, 182
critical realism, 168

demography of suicide, in England
      and Wales, 144–6
developmental studies of suicide,
      142
disciplinary power, 69
distribution of suicide, 9–10
double hermeneutic, and suicide,
      54–9
double life, of suicide, 34, 36
Douglas, J.D., 3, 177
   The Social Meanings of Suicide,
      18–23
dual paradigms approach, 42–5
Dumit, J., 68, 69
Duneier, M., 46
Durkheim, E., 3, 28–9, 144, 177
   Suicide: A Study in Sociology,
      8–15

egoistic suicide, 10–11, 36, 159
emotional aspects, of suicide notes,
      109–10
England
   demography of suicide in, 144–6
   suicide prevention policy, 173–7
Esquirol, 9

ethical research, 51–2
ethnographic approaches, to files and to life-course, 66–70
ethnomethodology, 26
evidence-based interventions, for suicide prevention, 179
experiences, and suicide, 111–12
  case studies, 115–16, 120–1, 125–6, 129–30

family breakdown, 156
family of suicidal person, 142
family problems, 153, 165
family society, and suicide, 11
fatherhood, 163
female suicides, 156
  see also gender
financial worries, 56
Foucault, M., 68
Freud, S., 143, 162
  psycho-analysis, 142
funerals, suicide notes on, 101–2

Gell, A., 83, 94
gender
  and relationship breakdown, 158–64
    murder and attempted murder, 160
    over-dependence, 161
    punishment, 160–1
    separation from children, 162–4
    sexual jealousy, 161–2
  identities and practices, 183
  suicide by, 149
  see also masculinities
Giddens, A., 35, 58, 159
  New Rules of Sociological Method, 31
good death, 96

health services, 180–2
history of suicide study, 8
Hjelmeland, H., 88
holistic responses, 183

identities of the deceased, 65–84, 183
immigrant populations, 33
insecure attachment, 140–1, 151
interactionism, 23, 24, 39
interpretivism, 39
interviews
  with eye witnesses, 49
  with relatives and friends, 49

Jamison, K.R., 38
Jones, E., 145

Klinenberg, E., 45, 46
Knizek, E.L., 88

Laub, J.H., 136, 137, 138
life-course, 66–70, 180
  criminology, 136
  ethnographic approaches to, 66–70
  social bonds and, 136–8

Maginot Lines, 38
masculinities, 61–2, 117, 122, 143, 161, 162, 163, 183
McCarthy Veach, P., 88
medical scientists, reports by, 70
medical specialists, reports by, 70
mental illness, suicide of people with, 175–6, 178
methodological pluralism, 41
mid-life, 148, 154–7, 165
Moat, R., 133, 134, 135, 166
model of others, 140
model of self, 140
morality, 69
murder and attempted murder, 160
murder-suicides, 133, 135, 160
mutual knowledge, 58

narrative therapy, 183
National Suicide Prevention Strategy for England, 173–5, 181, 182
naturalism, 43
nonfoundationalist realism, 168n9

objectivism, 43
official statistics, 21, 33
older people, 157–8
ontological hopelessness, 43
ordering of death, 68
oriental groups, 15
other-blame, 87

paradigm wars, 39–41
paramedics, as witnesses, 50
pathology reports, 50
personal disorganisation, and
    suicide, 17, 18
personhood, 65
Pescosolido, B.A., 30
physicians, reports by, 70
police officers, as witnesses, 50
possessions distribution, in suicide
    notes, 102–3
post-Durkheimian sociological
    theories, 20
post-mortem reports, 71–2
preliterate groups, 15
Prior, L., 68
prisoners, 183
private experiences, and suicide,
    14
psychiatric reports, 50–1
psychoanalysis, 136, 138–44
psychological autopsy, 47, 109
psychological reports, 35, 50–1
public, as witnesses, 50

quantitative/qualitative divide, 39,
    42–5

rebirth, 159
reflexive dimension, 22
relationship breakdown, 53, 54,
    56, 98, 155, 156, 171,
    178–9
religion, and suicide, 11
repertoires of action, 107, 108,
    112–13
  case studies, 113–31
  cognitive filters, 110
  concept of, 109–10

reports
  by medical scientists, medical
      specialists and physicians, 70
  on deceased person
    as corpse, 70–2
    as patient, 72–5
reproduced practice, suicide as a
    form of, 169–70
retaliatory abandonment, 159
reunion, 159
revenge, 159
Riles, A., 67–8

Sampson, R.J., 136–8
Sanger, S., 88
Schneidman, E., 86
scientism, 39
secure attachment, 140, 153
secure base, 139, 140
self-blame, 87
Silverman, D., 41
situated choice, 137
social anthropology, 94
social bonds, and life-course, 136–8
social circumstances of suicide,
    149–51
social context of suicide, across
    life-course, 151–8
  mid-life gendered patterns, 154–7
  older people in decline, 157–8
  young people in crisis, 153–4
social isolation, 144
social nomads, 138
social relationships, 131, 170–1
  children, 179–80
  partners, 178–9
socio-economic factors, and suicide
    prevention, 175
sociological autopsy approach, 38,
    45–7, 149
  limitations of, 59, 63, 174
sociology of suicide, 7–37, 54–5, 94,
    169
  divisions and oppositions, 30–6
status integration theory, 30
stimulus-response model of
    causation, 107

structuration theory, 31, 32, 137, 170
structure–agency interplay, 137
subtle realism, 168
suicide inquest files, 66–70
suicide notes, 48, 80–2
  emotional aspects, 109–10
  intendation, 100–1
    funerals, 101–2
    general material and practical aspects, 101
    possessions distribution, 102–3
  as social documents, 85
  social science perspective, 89–100
suicide prevention, 168, 172
  national strategies, 172–7, 185
  policies, 172, 173–7
suicidology, 2, 3, 4, 7, 24, 35, 42, 45, 88, 178, 183

text message, 91–2
types of suicide, 10

under-reporting of suicides, 52

values and beliefs, and suicide, 112
  case studies, 116–17, 122, 126, 130–1
variable analysis, 39

Wales, 144–6
  demography of suicide in, 144–6
war, and suicide, 29
Western culture, 22
witness statements, 75–80
women, 156
working models, 139
work-related problems, 154

youth suicide, 142, 153

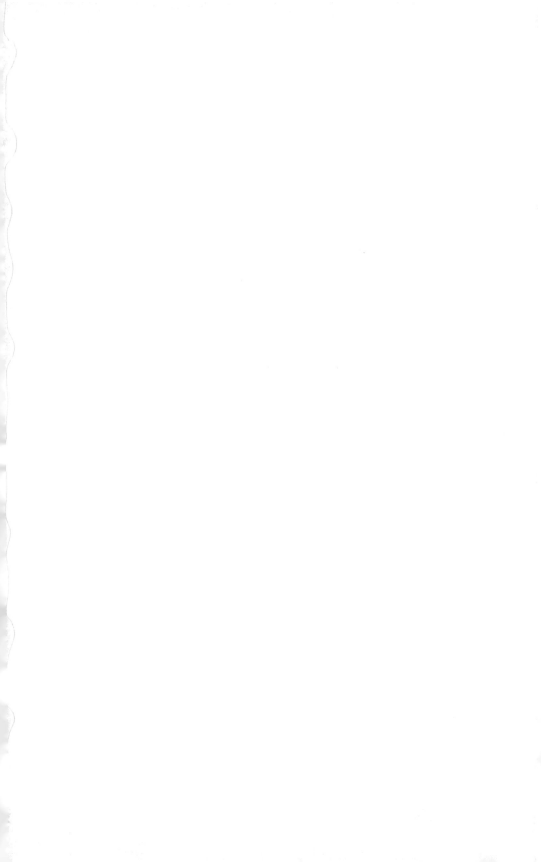